The process of
planning nursing care

A THEORETICAL MODEL

FAY LOUISE BOWER, R.N., B.S., M.S.N.
Associate Professor of Nursing and Associate Project Director of
Curriculum Revision, Department of Nursing, California State
University, San Jose, San Jose, California

Illustrated

THE C. V. MOSBY COMPANY

Saint Louis 1972

To:

Bob, my devoted husband, whose patience
and encouragement made it possible for
me to write.

Carol, my daughter, who cooked and cleaned
to free me from mundane chores.

David, my son, who kept asking, "How's
the book coming?"

Dennis, my son, who stayed clear of the
whole project.

Tom, my littlest angel, who never knew why
mother was always at the typewriter.

John, my son-in-law, who helped Carol
help me.

F. L. B.

Preface

Traditionally nurses have functioned autonomously in areas of health care other than those designated as the legal and professional responsibility of the physician. With a growing need for an extension of health services to great numbers of people, this independent role of the nurse is being extended. Pediatric nurse specialists and nurse midwives, to name just two, are examples of this extended role. Skill in independent judgment and the ability to assume responsibility for primary health care are expected of the nurse. Concomitant to this extended role is the expanded responsibility now being expected of the nurse. With a greater number and a greater variety of health workers involved as members of the health team, nurses are expected to include managerial and supervisory skills in their repertoire of behaviors. To compound the issue of change in role is the demand by the public for quality care. "Meeting needs" and "planning comprehensive care" are terms often expressed. But how is the nurse, busy adapting to an expanding and extended role, to develop skill in planning comprehensive and individualized care? It is the purpose of this book to help nurses develop increased skill in decision making as the process of planning care. With practice all nurses can increase their ability to make critical and astute decisions that have a high probability of success.

A second and equally important goal of this book is to present a theoretical framework for nurses that will enable them to plan holistic care, to plan care that meets the needs of the person as he responds holistically to his environment. The concepts of holism, stress response, wellness, and homeostasis are discussed and united to form a theoretical model for the identification of nursing problems. I hope that this holistic approach will enable the nurse to view the individual as a unique and dynamic system and that care can be planned to meet the needs and problems of the individual as he responds in a holistic manner to his environment.

Throughout the book I have used the term "client" to refer to the recipient of nursing care. This word was chosen because it most adequately describes the person who needs or seeks the promotion of health and the prevention of illness. The term is used inclusively to identify persons needing nursing care who are found in a variety of settings and who are experiencing a multiplicity of health problems or needs.

This book is divided into five chapters. The first chapter presents an overview of the process of planning nursing care. The second chapter presents a philosophical approach for the implementation of the nursing process and culminates in a theoretical model. The third chapter demonstrates a practical use of the holistic model in the first two phases of the nursing process, assessment and problem identification. The fourth chapter develops in detail the process of making a decision, the third phase of the nursing process, and gives examples of its use in common nursing situations. The evaluative phase is also discussed in Chapter 4. Chapter 5 contains a discussion of nursing care plans, their evolution, purpose, and content.

Without the support and encouragement of colleagues and the inspiration of students, this book could not have been completed. To them I am eternally grateful. Special thanks go to Miss Em Olivia Bevis, who reviewed the final manuscript.

Fay Louise Bower

Contents

The process of planning nursing care
A THEORETICAL MODEL

INTRODUCTION

Planned nursing care is the basis for nursing practice. Planning care is a systematic and complex process. Adequate planning involves not only knowledge of man and his adaptive behaviors but also a means of applying that knowledge to the promotion and maintenance of maximum health regardless of the environmental circumstances. Nursing has the unique property of operating in a highly generalistic manner; the breadth and scope of the nursing role exhibits no well-defined or agreed-upon parameter for health care. Concepts, theories, principles, and laws derived from the physical, behavioral, and social sciences serve as reference areas for the development of planned care as nurses collaborate with other disciplines in the delivery of health care. Because nursing focuses on individual need and assumes responsibility for total health care, nurses are faced with the task of planning care that is individualized and is concerned with the *total* health needs of the individual.

Never has the demand for quality and quantity of health care been at such a premium. Never has the role of the nurse been so challenged or been exposed to so much change as it is today. For example:

1. The number of eligible and interested persons demanding health care has increased.
2. Advances in medical technology have provided new and sophisticated tools for diagnosis and treatment.
3. The increased cost of hospitalization has promoted the continued growth of community-centered follow-up care, which emphasizes promotion of health rather than cure of illness.
4. Government funding for construction and health programs has increased the availability of health care.
5. The increasing number of paramedical and ancillary personnel entering the health scene, such as aides, orderlies, technologists, and practical nurses, has placed more and more emphasis on the managerial skills of the nurse.
6. Expanding use of self and role with increased need for nurses with

higher education has provided a basis for creative expansion of the nurse's role.

7. A shortage of physicians with a concomitant shift of responsibility for health care to the nurse has created an expanded role for the nurse.

8. Above all, the complex and rapidly changing social conditions with their accompanying changes of attitudes and values have produced community, family, and interpersonal problems that need identification and alleviation.

FACTORS THAT INFLUENCE THE PLANNING OF NURSING CARE
Increased demand for health care

Since health is now considered a fundamental right for all, there has been an increase in the number of individuals seeking health care. Membership in group insurance plans and federal and state-supported health plans have also increased the number of persons eligible for health care. Most employers provide their employees with the opportunity to purchase group health insurance. Through television, radio, and the newspapers, optimal health is promoted and prevention of illness is emphasized. The population explosion, which is the result of an upswing of births, a decrease in deaths, and an increase in life expectancy, has brought with it an increase in the number of persons needing health care. And along with longevity comes an increase in chronic problems, which means a need for long-term care. This increase in the number of persons seeking health care results in the need for more and better-prepared health professionals and health facilities that are used more efficiently and effectively.

Not only are more nurses needed, but better use of the nurse's skills is essential. The recipient of health care is smarter, more sophisticated, and more critical of things as they are and more insistent on an adequate response to his health needs than ever before. He demands to be involved in his care and he is determined to build a better life and achieve new goals. Nurses must respond to these expectations by planning adequate and effective individualized nursing care.

Technological advances

Technological advances have greatly affected health care. Radiology, electronic monitoring, advancements in surgery, diagnostic computer analysis, and chemotherapy have improved diagnosis and increased the individual's chances for optimum health. Organ transplants increase man's life expectancy and early diagnostic tests for malignant disease prevent destruction of tissues and also prolong life. Easy and accessible methods for early detection of abnormalities alert the physician and the nurse to impending health problems. Many of these technological advances directly affect nurses. Monitoring equipment frees the nurse from direct observation of the individual and yet increases responsibility. Nurses interpret the findings, operate the equipment, and repair equipment malfunctions. The nurse's understanding of radiology is useful in protecting the client and others so that maximum benefit from radiological treatment can be realized. An understanding of the many diagnostic tests available that detect shifts in the vital chemical components of the body (such as urine test tape for pH, sugar, and protein) is essential if the nurse is to teach the individual self-care. Knowledge of pharmaceutical agents used in therapy is also essential if optimal relief for the client is to be reached with minimal untoward reaction.

Computers are also influencing nursing care. They not only act as information banks but also diagnose, analyze, evaluate, sort, and record health problems. In the hospital setting computers are being used to prepare staffing schedules, to compile medication lists that are printed out for each hour that medications are given, to prepare census reports, and to match patients' needs with the proper qualified personnel. Physicians feed their orders into a computer, where they are stored until retrieved by the nurse, the x-ray department, the diet kitchen, or any other department concerned with the client's care. At the punch of a key printouts are available to these respective departments, where the orders are then carried out.

In other agencies much of the routine paper work is done by computers. Storage and retrieval systems are being used for storing information about clients to be retrieved on a printout when needed. Programming a computer to do the routine paper work frees the nurse for direct client care. Relieved of such tasks, the nurse has time to develop the skills of assessment, priority setting, interpersonal communication, and delegation and to focus on the human being and his unique response to his situation.

Growth of extended-care facilities

The high cost of hospitalization has promoted the continued growth of community-centered outpatient care. At one time diagnostic tests were performed exclusively in the hospital. But with spiraling costs and an increasing number of persons seeking hospital care, more and more outpatient facilities are being utilized to accomplish such tasks. The duration of hospitalization has also shortened because of skyrocketing costs. Even with medical and hospital insurance the average individual cannot afford to stay in the hospital for long periods of time. Therefore many individuals complete their convalescence at home and may need supervision. Nurses are often the persons called upon to assume the follow-up care after diagnosis and to manage the convalescent phase.

Some of the shift from hospital care to outpatient care is the result of legislation. For example, the Landis-Petri-Short Act of 1969 in California shifted the responsibility of psychiatric care from the state to the county.

This shift has created changes in treatment philosophy and role function, particularly for the nurse. For those clients who can manage themselves, treatment occurs on an outpatient basis, with the nurse joining the other professionals as a therapist. Nurses, psychiatrists, psychologists, social workers, and occupational therapists form the treatment team that assesses, evaluates, and provides crisis intervention and psychotherapy. In other areas of the United States similar shifts from hospital care to outpatient care are occurring.

Patterns of nursing care

A major influence that has increased the nurse's responsibility and to some extent changed the role is the addition of ancillary and paramedical personnel to the nursing team. Individuals trained to specialize in particular therapies such as the occupational therapist, the inhalation therapist, and the speech therapist pool their talents to offer the best care to the client. Nurse's aides, licensed vocational nurses, orderlies, and psychiatric technicians are prepared to carry out the nursing care plan under the direction and supervision of the nurse. Skill in leadership, which includes ease of delegation and evaluation, is an essential characteristic of the nurse. With so many individuals involved in the delivery of nursing care, accurate and individualized client assessment is the key to the success of the care. Many different patterns of nursing care have been tried with varying success. The case approach, the functional approach, and the team approach are the three patterns of nursing care most often utilized.

The case approach to the delivery of nursing care is used when one-to-one contact is desired. The case approach is utilized in intensive care units and coronary care units and any specialized unit where expertise and close or prolonged observation and care are required; total care of the client is the responsibility of one person. Nurse counselors and therapists often relate on a one-to-one basis when helping an individual or a family work through interpersonal problems. Public health nurses use the case approach because their work load is comprised of families that they counsel toward behavioral change. Through anticipatory guidance, health teaching, and screening, they identify health problems and develop nursing interventions.

Another pattern of care often used is the functional approach. With this approach a particular duty or task is assigned to an individual; a duty that the individual is prepared to meet. Many individuals are involved in the care of one client, each carrying out a portion of the total nursing care. The danger of such an approach is the fractionalization of care. To avoid this danger, the nurse acts as coordinator and interpreter of the nursing care.

Perhaps the best method of delivery of nursing care is the team approach in which a group of people works together to meet the needs of a number of clients. The team approach is based on the philosophy that optimal use of all personnel is possible when the preparation and talents of each team member are matched with the client's assessed needs. With this approach all personnel have contact with the clients and have a share in planning and providing nursing care. Although many people are involved in the nursing care, the emphasis is on the individual's needs and not on tasks to be accomplished. The client benefits by receiving the best service each team member is capable of rendering. The nurse team leader acts as coordinator, supervisor, and resource person to the team. Unlike the functional method of assignment, the team approach maintains the totality of the client, while enabling each member of a nursing group to utilize his particular area of interest and skill.

Although all three approaches demand the nurse's ability to assess and plan care, each method requires a different type of planning. Case method assignment requires the nurse alone to plan and implement nursing care. The functional method requires that the nurse collaborate with other members of the nursing team to plan care, but limits the members' contacts with one another. When the team approach is employed, planning becomes the team's responsibility; team members become involved in assessing needs, identifying problems, and deciding on interventions.

Physician distribution

One of the major reasons that the nurse's role is changing and expanding is the shortage of physicians. Many counties in many states, particularly rural communities, do not have a physician. Because large metropolitan areas with high-density population attract physicians, many rural areas go without adequate physician coverage. In such events, primary care is often dispensed by nurses. Even in the densely populated areas, physicians are delegating responsibilities for health care to nurses so that they can make better use of their time and talents as physicians. Such titles as Pediatric Nurse Practitioner, Clinical Nurse Specialist, and Nurse Psychotherapist have been coined to describe the expanded role of the nurse. Time and space do not allow for a detailed discussion of the many opportunities available for the nurse, but the situation has become impressive and is a major influence on the planning of nursing care.

Regardless of the title, the nurse's role is changing and expanding, with growing responsibility. Many of the traditional tasks and decisions that physicians performed are now the concern of nurses. With the expanding role comes the need to plan care that reflects this added responsibility.

Rapidly changing social and environmental conditions

Rapidly changing social conditions are also affecting nursing care. The shorter work week and earlier retirement have produced more leisure time and a subsequent need for recreational planning. Crowded ghetto living with its inherent health problems has precipitated riots and other acts of personal violence. Immediate treatment, as well as prevention of such disasters, is necessary and is an integral part of nursing care planning. Increased community interest and concern have created political and economic pressure groups, which are determined to provide better housing and living conditions for the vast number of poverty groups. Revised welfare programs and comprehensive health care based on need rather than on economic situation are occurring as a result of federal legislation.

Health care workers have long been aware of the fact that personal and environmental health are inseparable. Dr. Roger O. Egeberg of the Department of Health, Education, and Welfare recently ranked the nation's most serious health problems, in order of priority, as follows:

1. Health care delivery
2. Population control and cleanup of the environment
3. Need for support of basic research
4. Alcoholism and other addictive diseases

More and more legislative effort is being focused on solving environmental problems. Results of this emphasis can be seen in the Clean Air Act and the National Water Quality Act. Legislation such as this endeavors to protect natural resources, to conserve and protect beauty, and to control air and water pollution and demonstrates the community's concern to develop solutions to health problems.

The world population explosion is a major concern to everyone interested in health. The population explosion poses a serious threat to the world food supply. Crowding in high-density areas has created water pollution and waste disposal problems. Air, land, water, and food are not unlimited; and the maintenance of the quality and quantity of these resources has become a tremendous task. To combat overpopulation birth control information, sex education in the schools, and legalized abortion will be needed. Nurses will be prime innovators and disseminators of this information.

Water is a critical environmental problem because of shortage and pollution. Expanding population and an expanded use of water for farming and industry are causing an acute water shortage. Depletion of underground water reserves allows brine to seep into underground water reserves and renders the water useless for drinking, industry, and irrigation. The increased use of detergents continues to pollute the subterranean water supplies. Industrial pollution not only increases the temperature of our natural water resources and kills the fish, but also adds to reserves contaminants that pollute the water for human consumption. Spraying, crop dusting, fumigation, and storage of insecticides continue to create health problems, such as food contamination, accidental contact with humans, and contamination of streams and other water supplies. More federal legislation and control is needed to effectively stop or prevent further pollution. Much public education is needed to protect the public and prevent disease.

Air pollution has increased to the point of great concern. High-density smog over large geographical areas caused by transportation and industrial waste cause death of some trees and small plants, decreased rainfall, and decreased food production. There is an increase of lung disease (emphysema, bronchitis, asthma, and cancer) and an increase in chronic and acute eye inflammation. Some action leading to solution of the air pollution problem is already under way. Some states have automobile emission control laws. Electric and steam cars; monorail systems; atomic, tidal, and solar power for the electricity industry; and larger transportation devices are just a few of the potential solutions to air pollution already being considered and tried.

Modern transportation and the developing tastes of people for a wider variety of nonlocal foods have caused an increase in food-borne illnesses. Changes in production and processing of foods and food treatment with chemicals both in the fields and in the processing plants have detrimental effects on human and animal health.

Drug use and abuse have pyramided to the point of major concern. The rapidity of technological change and the ever-spiraling pace with which humans must adjust constitute a major factor for the use of alcohol and other psyche-altering drugs. More public facilities and centers for research and treatment for drug users are needed. Nurses again have a leading role to play in this fight to preserve health.

Changing family life styles

Changes in the community health milieu often have their genesis in changing family life styles. Changes in family configuration and role function are the result of a world in social and cultural flux. Before the industrial revolution the extended family lived either with or close to the primary family. The health and welfare of either was the concern of both. But with the escalation of technology, employment opportunities severed the primary family from the extended family. Federally financed care for the aged, supplied through the Social Security Act of 1934 and greatly expanded in the Medicare Act of 1969, has shifted the responsibility for health care from the family to the government. An increase in health professionals is not only needed to meet the growing needs of a generation that lives longer but also for those aged persons who no longer have their extended family members as their prime source of health care.

Communal family structure presents another type of changing family configuration that affects the planning and delivery of nursing care. Those who live in communes are often distrustful of established health care facilities and health personnel yet are in great need of health education. Nurses need to be aware of and understand how to offer informal, nonjudgmental, and youth-oriented care that is acceptable and compatible with their mores, values, and life style. Planning for this kind of approach requires that nurses be sensitive and alert to their own values and attitudes and be able to devise a method of "reaching out."

Other changes are occurring within the traditional family unit. High divorce rates and the increasing equality of women in both status and opportunity have increased the number of women employed outside the home. In many instances management of the home, child rearing, and income are the shared responsibilities of the husband and the wife, with an accompanying blurring of roles. Whereas it once was easy for a child to identify with the father as the "bread winner" and the "head of the house," now, because of circumstances such as divorce, there is no definitive father-role model. The result of such role blurring and lack of role models is often evidenced in the child's inability to clearly establish his own identity.

Even more important is the "communication gap" that exists in many families. An inability to exchange and accept different ideas, values, and attitudes has created strained family relationships and anxiety for both parent and child. Nurses have endless opportunities to help families bridge the communication gap and to prevent family breakup and promote healthy parent-child relations.

Social, environmental, and family changes are reflected in the changing role of the community health nurse. According to Freeman:

> Community health nursing is seen as a population-based obligation, realized through a multidisciplinary, ecologically oriented effort and utilizing concepts and skills that derive both from generic nursing and from public health practices. It focuses on nursing the community in contradiction to nursing in the community. Family nursing care is seen as an essential aspect of health care of the population, and the community health nurse's responsibility is seen as encompassing but not being limited to this aspect of the program.[1]

Planning nursing care that puts these concepts into action is not limited to the care of persons outside the hospital. It is directed toward the population as a whole. It requires collaborative planning with other disciplines, involvement of the family in decisions, and skill in initiating nursing actions that are based on knowledge of sociocultural patterns and the theories of learning and motivation.

---

[1]Freeman, Ruth B.: Community health nursing practice, Philadelphia, 1970, W. B. Saunders Company, p. 111.

Chapter

1

PLANNING INDIVIDUALIZED NURSING CARE
TO MEET CHANGING NEEDS

Reality, as it is given to us in wonder, presents itself to us as something having a dignity, worth, meaning, or value which calls forth admiration and appreciation.

Sam Keen, *Apology for Wonder*[1]

OVERVIEW

Planning nursing care that will meet the needs of people in a constantly changing milieu demands that the nurse be able to analyze, synthesize, and organize an incredible amount of data. To accomplish this involved and complex task and to preserve the individuality of the person or family, nurses assess health needs, determine nursing interventions, refer persons to appropriate professionals or agencies, and establish priorities in nursing care. Nursing care planning, then, is a decision-making process that requires a systematic and comprehensive approach. The purpose of this chapter is twofold: (1) to give an overview of the process of planning nursing care, and (2) to demonstrate the use of decision making as a process in planning nursing care. Subsequent chapters will handle each phase of the decision-making process in detail.

PROCESS OF PLANNING NURSING CARE

The process of planning nursing care is a systematic step-by-step method of selecting an action or actions to reach a desired goal. It is a decision-making process. It includes both cognitive and activity components. The goal of planned nursing care is to help the individual or the family (the client) reach a state of high-level wellness.[2]

Nursing care planning can be divided into four phases: (1) assessment, (2)

---

[1] Keen, Sam: Apology for wonder, New York, 1969, Harper & Row, Publishers.
[2] Dunn, Halbert L.: High-level wellness, Virginia, 1961, R. W. Beatty, Ltd., p. 4.

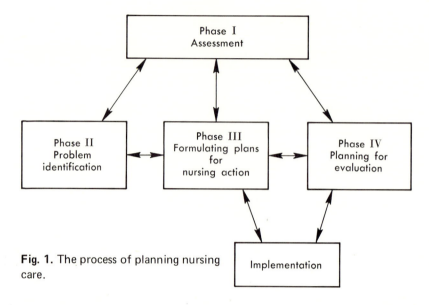

Fig. 1. The process of planning nursing care.

problem identification, (3) formulation of a plan, and (4) planning for evaluation. Each phase is separate from the others but interdependent with the others. The whole process is dynamic, since data from one phase can alter or support the other phases.

Decisions are continually being made by every individual. It is impossible to go through a day without making some kind of decision. Some decisions occur by chance or by repetition of an action because it worked before. For the best results, however, decisions should be thought out, critically analyzed, and astutely conceived, since the act of decision making involves choosing from alternatives[3] and nursing care planning is a decision-making process. Nurses cannot assess a situation, identify a problem, or determine an intervention without considering alternative approaches for the best way of solving a problem or meeting a need.

ASSESSMENT

Assessment is the first phase in planning nursing care. It consists of the collection of data from many sources, which are then classified, analyzed, and summarized to determine nursing problems or needs.

Data collection is time consuming but is an absolutely essential part of problem identification. It involves astute observation, purposeful listening, a broad knowledge of human behavior, and an understanding of what needs to be known and where to obtain that information. Individuality in nursing care

[3] Bross, I. D. J.: Design for decision, New York, 1953, The Macmillan Company.

can be expected if the data collected are accurate, complete, and properly analyzed.

Data can be collected from many sources. The client's past history, his health and family history, his knowledge of the present health situation, his expectations of care, and any baseline information (vital statistics) that currently affects the individual are areas that contribute to the assessment. After data are collected, the nurse organizes the material into related groups from which inferences, speculations, and interpretations of the client's health needs or problems are made. Although data collection is the first step in planning nursing care, it also occurs throughout the nursing process. New data about the client or situation may be obtained during any phase of the nursing process. On the other hand, the other phases of the nursing care process cannot be performed in a meaningful or purposeful manner unless they are based on data pertinent to the situation.

In any nursing care process there are facts that are immediately available to the nurse and areas that need to be discovered. For example, consider the following situation:

> When making rounds on a medical unit, a nurse looks in on a middle-aged gentleman who is sitting in a chair eating his lunch. He is in the hospital with a diagnosis of acute myocardial infarction. His wife is eating lunch with him as he convalesces. Suddenly the gentleman turns pale, gasps, and slumps forward.

From this situation the nurse knows: (1) a gentleman is convalescing from a myocardial infarction; (2) he is middle aged; (3) he is eating his lunch; (4) he turns pale, gasps, and slumps forward. With this information two possible inferences can be made. The gentleman is either choking on something he is eating (inference from the fact that he is seen eating) or he is having a heart attack (inference from the fact that he is convalescing from a previous heart attack and that he is middle aged. Middle-aged men experience a high incidence of heart attack). Further data collection is necessary before the nurse can define the gentleman's problem and before action can be taken. Obviously the nurse should examine the gentleman's airway for food particles, observe him for other clues, and question his wife for more information.

Nurses use a variety of sources for data collection and all are necessary for the planning of personalized comprehensive nursing care. When these data are sorted into various categories, it is possible to identify the client's or the family's nursing problems.

Problem identification

In order to solve a problem it is necessary that the nurse recognizes that a problem exists. It seems redundant to say this, but one reason nursing care often fails to satisfy the needs of the client is that nurses do not recognize nursing problems.

Problem situations vary. Some problems are overt, some covert.[4] Overt problems are problems that are easily recognized. Covert problems are problems that are difficult to identify either because of a lack of data, an overlay of other problems, or a lack of objectivity. These problems need to be discovered. In either case the process of problem identification is the same; however, since covert problems are more difficult to identify, the nurse needs to gather all available data and employ particular care in systematically sifting out the problem.

Problem identification begins with an identification of the client's needs. Once data have been collected and analyzed, these data are utilized to determine what needs the client presents. Information from observation, interview, and ongoing appraisal is arranged into categories for analysis. If, on analysis, the data indicate unmet needs or blocked goals, then a problem exists. By definition a problem is an interruption in the individual's ability to meet a need; it is a difficulty or a perplexity that requires resolution. Problems exist when there is no straight-line action possible.[5] This means a progression of events toward need gratification has been interrupted, altered, or disturbed; in some way need gratification is not clearly or discernibly evident. Abraham Maslow has identified man's basic needs, in order of hierarchy, as follows:

1. Hunger, thirst, sex, and survival
2. Safety, self-preservation, security
3. Belongingness and love
4. Social esteem and self-respect
5. Self-actualization[6]

Certain factors influence the extent to which each individual is able to meet his basic needs—factors such as age, culture, emotions, environment, intellectual capacity, sex, disease, and the individual's ability to cope. Whenever an individual or a family is not able to meet basic needs, requires assistance with meeting a need, or does not recognize an unmet need a problem exists. Nursing problems arise from those unmet needs that are within the context of health. In other words, if any unmet need impinges on the individual's or the family's ability to maintain or improve health and the nurse can be of assistance, a nursing problem exists. Nursing problems also occur when a person is trying to meet needs in an inappropriate manner.

---

[4] Brown, Martha, and Fowler, Grace: Psychodynamic nursing: a biosocial orientation, ed. 4, Philadelphia, 1971, W. B. Saunders Company, p. 14.

[5] MacDonald, Frederick J.: Educational psychology, ed. 2, Belmont, 1969, Wadsworth Publishing Co., Inc., p. 253.

[6] Maslow, Abraham: Toward a psychology of being, New York, 1962, D. Van Nostrand Co., Inc., pp. 19-24.

Data analysis may point up problems that are outside the realm of nursing, problems that are the concern of the physician, social worker, or some other member of the health team. For instance, a community health nurse, while visiting a family, discovers a person who presents the symptoms of pulmonary tuberculosis. In such a case the nurse must refer the person to a physician for diagnosis and treatment. But it is the nurse's job to report the health problem to the proper authorities to protect the rest of the community and to provide health supervision and follow-up care for the sick individual and his family. The signs and symptoms, mode of entry, and means of transmission of pulmonary tuberculosis will need to be explained to the family by the nurse. The nurse will also need to evaluate the family's nutrition and other health practices to determine if they are adequate and do not contribute to the health problem.

Sometimes a health problem is the concern of many health professionals. Each will handle the situation in a different way. The differences are in terms of each professional's expertise—the type of service offered by each. Of major importance is the collaborative nature of nursing care with other members of the health care system to provide safe, effective prevention and treatment.

Stating the nursing problem

The statement of the nursing problem defines the nursing goal. If nursing problems are the result of an individual's inability to meet his needs or of inappropriate need gratification, then the statement of the problem tells what should be accomplished. For example, if the client's need is for sleep but sleep is blocked by a severe cough, the statement of the problem would be "how to relieve the client's cough to provide sleep." The objective of the nursing care is to provide the client with sleep by relieving his cough. Nursing actions will determine the method for relieving the cough.

The essential consideration in stating a nursing problem is to communicate the intent or goal to those engaged in working with the problem, principally the client, the nursing team members, and others involved in the care of the client. Some nurses prefer to identify client needs and state the problem as a statement of need. If one accepts the definition of a nursing problem as an unmet need, it is better to separate the need from the problem and state each accordingly.

PRIORITY SETTING

Priority setting refers to the act of giving preferential attention to one thing over competing alternatives.[7] After the needs of the client and the

---

[7]Merriam-Webster, A.: Webster's third new international dictionary (unabridged), vol. II Chicago, 1966, William Benton, p. 1804.

resultant nursing problems have been identified, the nurse should rank them in order of priority. This phase of the problem-identification process is vital because some nursing problems are more critical than others and require ranking so that those with the greatest urgency, the greatest threat, or the gravest consequences will be considered first. Priority setting is a device that requires the nurse to classify and sort (1) life-threatening problems from ones of lesser importance, (2) short-term immediate problems from long-term problems, (3) conflicting goals to determine which goal to meet and when. Even with the best of intentions nurses cannot possibly meet all the client's needs or help him solve all his health problems. Priority setting enables the nurse to organize and plan care that meets those needs and solves those problems that are most urgent, and to consider ways and means of handling the problems of lesser urgency. Priority setting does not negate the importance of the lower-priority problems; it simply puts problems into a realistic framework for consideration and solution. Many factors affect priority setting: values, policy, money, time, and goals. These factors often determine the priority of a nursing problem.

Criteria for priority setting

All of the nursing problems of the client, family, or community must be considered when setting priorities. A criterion for setting priorities enables the nurse to determine a hierarchy of importance. Criteria of hierarchy should include the consideration of (1) those problems that threaten the life, dignity, and integrity of the individual, family, or community; (2) those problems that threaten to destructively change the individual, family, or community; and (3) those problems that affect the normal developmental growth of the individual, family, or community.

Health problems that affect the life of an individual or his family take first priority. In a client with cardiac arrest the nurse moves to maintain an open airway and to ventilate the lungs before considering measures to improve the heart's action.[8] Problems that threaten the family unit's *integrity* take precedence over other types of family problems. When a father's alcoholism is the precipitating cause of conflict and possible family breakdown, this problem gets preferential attention over other health problems, such as the need for the children's immunizations and dental care. Although the nurse will certainly plan to handle these last two health needs, prime consideration goes to the preservation of the family unit. The same is true of community health problems. A major outbreak of smallpox would receive high priority, since such an epidemic could seriously affect the whole community.

Health problems that threaten to destructively change the individual or

---

[8]Jude, James R. and Blam, James O.: Fundamentals of cardiopulmonary resuscitation, Philadelphia, 1965, F. A. Davis Co., pp. 16-18.

the family take second priority. Changes in a person's personality that result in his withdrawal into a world of subjective construction fall into this category. Because these changes remove the individual from social contact, split him from reality, and limit his capacity to live a healthy productive life, they are classified as destructive changes. Abnormal cell growth that destroys organs, metabolic imbalance that disrupts normal functioning, and the loss of a body part, which creates a poor self-image, can also destructively change a person.

Breakdowns in communication, chronic degenerative disease processes, and traumatic injury, to name a few, can alter the lives of family members and ultimately lead to destructive changes in families. A rise in the use of illegal drugs, with an accompanying rise in crime, can destroy a community. Nurses as well as other interested professionals will give high priority to problems that threaten to destroy the family or the community.

Problems that affect the normal developmental growth of an individual take third priority. An individual who is nutritionally deprived cannot reach his maximum growth potential and therefore may develop a health problem. A family who, for any number of reasons, is unable to function as a unit to offer support to any of its growing members is not a thriving developing unit. A community that is hampered by a lack of funds and a lack of creative ideas or innovative programs does not progress, grow, or adapt to changing social needs. Problems like these can severely forestall or block growth; and although they do not take the highest priority, if they are not given attention they will eventually become serious threats to the life of the individual and the integrity of the family or the community.

Nurses need to consider ways of structuring nursing actions so that several levels of problems can be solved simultaneously. As high-level problems are met, lower-level problems shift upward. Thus, nurses must be aware of the potential for solving problems at each level and of the need to be formulating plans for more than one level of problems. Although this may seem difficult, with careful evaluation it becomes evident that certain nursing actions handle more than one level of problems. For example, Mr. Jones, an elderly man with gout, is in pain and is lonely. The nurse decides to relieve his pain by repositioning his foot and by administering an analgesic. This nursing action not only provides comfort for Mr. Jones but, because the nurse stayed a few minutes after administering the medication to talk with Mr. Jones, it also relieves his loneliness.

The degree to which the client or the family is involved in priority setting depends on several things. The condition of the client or family, an understanding of the situation, and a desire to be involved dictate when involvement can be expected. Client or family involvement in priority setting is desired because participation is not only a motivating behavior but it also demonstrates a certain amount of commitment to the outcome of the planning. Some persons are anxious to be involved in their plan of care, whereas others are happy to place the decisions in the hands of professionals. A cardinal rule in planning care and in setting priorities is to allow the client to make the decision of whether to be involved or not. No matter how "good" it might seem to have the client included in the planning of nursing care, nothing is more disastrous than a situation in which the client is forced to make decisions he plainly does not want to or cannot make.

Setting priorities for groups

The nurse may have several clients or families to attend to and therefore will need to set further priorities. The criteria for setting priorities when faced with more than one client or a group of clients are:
1. Safety
    A. Severity of health problems
    B. Potential for recovery
    C. Attainment of high-level wellness
2. Efficiency—time needed by client, nurse, or health team
3. Cost—expense in money and energy to client, nurse, agency, society
4. Receptivity to care

Those individuals or families that are in crisis situations receive priority over those with long-term chronic problems because the probability of return to a normal functioning and a productive life is higher in crisis situations than in chronic long-term situations.[9] Children, pregnant women, and acutely ill clients get preferential treatment over long-term emphysemic geriatrics and chronic schizophrenics. The prognosis for return to society and to a productive life is greater with the former than with the latter, since their potential for recovery and attainment of optimal health is higher.

The nurse's available time for care is a strong determinant in setting priorities. Some clients need little of the nurse's time, whereas others demand lengthy contact. When considering a priority ranking of all the clients within a group for nursing care, the nurse estimates how much nursing time is available and how much time each client will need. Some nurses prefer to care for the client who needs the most time first. Others leave the time-consuming client until last. The decision often rests with the nurse's own particular ability to organize and plot out economical use of time. Each nurse has idiosyncracies about how time is best used. What is important is that manpower is expensive and should not be wasted but should be utilized to the best advantage for safe and quality delivery of care. Setting priorities of care can help this occur.

One reason group teaching and group therapy have become so popular is

---

[9]Caplan, Gerald: An approach to community mental health, New York, 1961, Grune & Stratton, Inc., pp. 39-46.

that they make more efficient use of time. Aside from the fact that group teaching and group therapy also provide the clients with a chance to gain from interaction with others, they also utilize the nurse's time more efficiently. Why teach ten clients individually about diabetic diets when one session with all ten could accomplish the same objective? Group work saves precious time that the nurse can easily use for some other purpose.

Time limits need not hamper the quality of nursing care. With proper evaluation of the client's needs, the best approach for the client's care and the best use of the nurse's time can be determined. When making assignments, the nurse needs to critically determine how best to delegate the nursing care. The intelligent use of nursing personnel to meet the needs of a group of clients assures quality care; this means that various nursing personnel are assigned those aspects of the client's care that they are best prepared to do. To plan care for the sole purpose of saving time is wasteful of manpower and unfair to the client; but to plan care *without* considering the time factor is also wasteful of manpower and unfair to the client, because the best use of the nurse's time is disregarded.

Susceptibility to disease or relapse play a part in determining priorities. Very young children and the aged are more susceptible to health problems than others in the population. Pregnant women, the malnourished, and those recovering from a health problem need close supervision and continued attention. Persons who have been in close contact with someone who has been sick deserve high priority to prevent further problems. These people are more susceptible because they are more prone to disease, less able to cope with problems, and are therefore in greater need of assistance.

Another kind of susceptibility that affects priority setting is receptivity. Some persons are more prone or more open to suggestion and help; they accept and desire help and are willing to carry out the nursing plan. Others are reluctant or resistant to help. For expediency the most receptive client should be given priority. However, this does not mean that the nurse should ignore those who are hesitant or who flatly reject nursing care. It means that the nurse should utilize the strengths and frailties of each individual in planning care so that each is accommodated appropriately. When the nurse handles the receptive client first, time is available for discovering why the others do not seek or accept nursing care. If the reverse method is used, that is, if the nurse gives priority to the person who is reluctant to accept or who rejects nursing care, time very likely will not be left for those who seek care and are eager for help.

Priority setting is a process that establishes a preferential order to the delivery of nursing care. It helps rule out those areas that need not be handled, as well as arrange the nursing problems in order of importance. Once the selection of problems to receive nursing attention has been made, planning for intervention begins.

PLANNING FOR NURSING INTERVENTION

A plan is a design for action. Nurses determine goals and articulate them in plans. Plans are formulated from decisions. Decisions guide action because they are the selected choices that actions follow.

Decision making is a complex behavior that requires the selection of a choice from many possibilities for the purpose of meeting a desired goal. Each choice or alternative is a possible way of attaining the goal. Each alternative has an expected effect or consequence when carried into action. For example, consider a situation in which a nurse in a hospital is faced with deciding what to do about a patient's pain. The patient is anxious, in pain, and has no order for pain medication. The nurse has the following alternative choices:

1. Try to comfort the patient by reducing his anxiety.
2. Reposition him.
3. Call his physician to obtain an order for medication.
4. Tell him, "I'm sorry I have no order for pain medication."

The consequences for alternative number 3 are:

1. The nurse may get the order.
2. The nurse may not be able to reach the physician.
3. The nurse may reach the physician and be denied an order for medication.

With each of the other alternative choices there are predictable consequences also.

Associated with the possible consequences of any alternative is the likelihood of the consequences occurring.[10] Certain information is required to determine the likelihood of any given consequence occurring. Facts, concepts, principles, and predictive theories are necessary in order to predict consequences and establish probability of occurrence. Nurses need a background in the behavioral sciences and the natural sciences, which they can assimilate and interpret to predict consequences and estimate probability of occurrence.

Probability can be expressed in two ways: in word form or in numerical symbolic form. Words such as high, medium, or low designate the relative value of a consequence. Probability of occurrence can be estimated by a scale of 0.10 to 1.00 with the lowest decimal number (0.10) representing very low probability. To determine the probability of a consequence the nurse estimates the likelihood of the consequence occurring and gives this occurrence a symbolic numerical figure. If the consequence always occurs it receives a numerical figure of 1.00. This means the consequence's probability of occurrence is 100% or ten times out of ten. However, if the consequence

---

[10]MacDonald, Frederick J.: Educational psychology, Belmont, 1965, Wadsworth Publishing Co., Inc., pp. 49-50.

occurs very seldom, say once or twice out of ten times, it then receives a probability of 0.10 or 0.20. A consequence that may or may not occur, one that has a questionable occurrence, receives a 0.50 probability; 0.50 probability refers to a 50/50 chance of occurrence. For the sake of clarity and uniformity, probability estimates can be classified into high probability occurrence (0.99 to 0.80), probable occurrence (0.79 to 0.60), questionable occurrence (0.59 to 0.50), low probability occurrence (0.49 to 0.30), and very low probability occurrence (0.29 to 0.10). The nurse is seeking the consequence with the highest probability of occurrence and is therefore looking for actions that have consequences that are rated 0.60 or over.[11] An example of the use of probability in the pain situation looks like this:

Alternative	*Consequence*	*Probability*
Call the physician	Get an order	0.75 (75%)
	Denied order	0.25 (25%)
	Unable to reach physician	0.50 (50%)

Some questionable actions, if tested—that is, taken to completion—produce higher probability of occurrence than estimated. It is of prime importance that the nurse remember that probability estimates are *estimates* of occurrence. Probability is a *tool* for helping the nurse make decisions. It is not a formula for decision making. Certainly nurses will differ in their estimates of probability, as they will differ in their approach to nursing care. There is no need, nor is it desirable, to unify nursing estimates. Decision making that is based on the consideration of the probability of consequences is designed to help each nurse critically analyze nursing actions, not to make all nurses act the same.

The value or desirability of any consequence also influences decision making.[12] Decisions are often based on judgments of the desirability of the expected outcome. The sources of these judgments are varied. Some are the result of a philosophy of life, some are derived from experience, some from preference, and some reflect the social and cultural mores.

Another dimension that helps the nurse make a decision when planning nursing actions is the consideration of the risk of the consequence to the client. Risk refers to danger or jeopardy to the client's life, safety, or well-being. Risk also involves consideration of legality, morality, and policy. Any nursing action must be evaluated in light of its possible risk to the nurse and the agency, as well as to the client.

Suppose a consequence of an action is highly probable and is desirable but poses a risk to the client. Consider again the patient in pain.

---

[11] Probability estimates will be discussed in depth in Chapter Five.
[12] MacDonald: Educational psychology, pp. 53-55.

The patient in pain is a 66-year-old man, first day postoperative after a right knee arthrotomy. The physician has an order on the patient's chart for morphine gr. 1/4 for pain relief every 4 hours. The nurse checks and discovers that the patient's respirations are 10 per minute and that he was medicated with morphine 2 hours ago.

The probability that the medication will relieve the pain if given now is high (0.95), but the risk to the patient is also high because of the depressive effect morphine has on respirations, which are already reduced. To give this man morphine for pain is very risky, therefore the nurse should consider other possible actions and their consequences. Refer to Fig. 2 for an illustration of this situation.

The action most likely chosen in Fig. 2 would be Approaches C and D. An analysis of all the possible nursing actions and their consequences rules out Approach A because it has a high-risk consequence in Consequence (2), and rules out Approach B because it has a high probability of occurrence with an undesirable value producing a high risk. Approaches C and D are good choices because Approach C has two consequences, (1) and (3), that are desirable, both have no apparent risk to the patient, and the probability of occurrence of both is over 0.50, or 50%. Only one consequence (2) is undesirable because of a moderate risk. But this consequence also has a questionable probability of occurrence (0.40). Approach D has one consequence that is desirable and without risk, with a probability of 0.70. The other consequence is undesirable

APPROACH	CONSEQUENCE(S)	PROB.	VALUE	RISK
A. Give morphine for pain relief	(1) will relieve pain	0.95	desirable	none
	(2) will decrease respirations	0.80	undesirable	high
	(3) will not relieve pain	0.05	undesirable	low
B. Not give morphine	(1) no pain relief	1.00	undesirable	high
C. Position patient and stay with him	(1) may relieve pain	0.60	desirable	none
	(2) may not relieve pain	0.40	undesirable	moderate
	(3) may decrease anxiety and thus reduce pain perception	0.50	desirable	none
D. Call doctor for change in medication	(1) may reach doctor and get new medication order	0.70	desirable	none
	(2) may reach doctor and not get new medication order	0.30	undesirable	moderate

Fig. 2. Selection of alternatives.

with moderate risk but with a lower probability of occurrence. Therefore Approaches C and D, when considered in totality, are apparently safe and effective approaches to try.

As demonstrated in the above example, a rule of decision making is to choose that action whose consequences have the highest probability of occurring and whose over-all values are high for the desired effect yet create the least risk to the client, nurse, or agency.

In some cases and usually in very critical situations, the value of the decision is determined by the risk. For instance, suppose the man with the pain in the above situation has a cardiac problem and is experiencing pain from a myocardial infarction and not from a first day postoperative arthrotomy. Under these circumstances Approaches B, C, and D are all inappropriate because with the changed situation they present undesirable value and high risk. Positioning will not relieve pain and calling for a change in pain medication wastes precious time. Prompt relief of pain is important, since pain intensifies shock, which is always present in some degree with myocardial infarction. Approach A is the only choice, since it will produce the desired effect. The risk of not giving the pain medication is greater than the risk of doing so. Concomitant to the administration of pain medication is the administration of oxygen. Such action could also be placed on the chart for consideration with an analysis of the consequence's probability of occurrence, value, and risk.

Rules of decision making based on the consideration of the probability, value, and risk of an action's consequences lack absolute validity. They have varying degrees of validity depending on many conditions. Validity is best obtained by evaluation. Once the action is carried out, the nurse gathers data from all available sources to determine if the nursing decision was valid, that is, did it accomplish the desired outcome.

To this point the decision-making process has been cognitive. Information and knowledge from many sources has enabled the nurse to plan for the nursing action. The fourth and final phase of the decision-making process is the evaluation of the nursing action. It is at this point that the nurse tests the effectiveness of the decision and the validity of the decision rule.

Evaluation

Each of the decisions that the nurse makes in formulating an action is hypothetical. Decisions show a relationship between a set of conditions and their effect. They assume a certain set of conditions and predict certain effects. In the fourth phase of decision making the nurse carries the plan into action and receives feedback about the effects of the decision so that an evaluation can be made. The feedback is utilized as new information to revise the plan when necessary. The nurse can plan and control the feedback to modify the plans for action.

Sources of feedback

Feedback from the nursing action originates from many sources. The nurse who carries out the action collects data about the intervention in much the same manner as was done earlier for the identification of the problem. Astute observation, purposeful listening, and open and direct communication give the nurse the needed information. After collecting the information the nurse sorts, classifies, and through deductive and inductive analysis, makes a judgment as to whether the action met the desired goal. The nurse also considers whether the action was economical of time, energy, and cost to self, agency, and client. An important source of feedback for evaluation consists of (1) the client's behavior, and (2) the client's verbalized subjective data. For instance, when the goal of the nursing action is relief of pain, evidence of comfort is sought. Observations of the client's position and facial expression coupled with his verbalized subjective feelings tell the nurse whether the client is comfortable. If the goal of the nursing action is to teach the client about his health problem, then evidence of learning is needed. Data collected from the learner about what was received and how it was interpreted tell the nurse whether learning occurred. If the learner repeatedly demonstrates the desired change, the nurse has evidence that he has learned.

Many nursing actions are interdependent and are designed in collaboration with the other members of the health team. Collaborative planning and evaluation allow for a wider variety of ideas to be considered. Plans have a greater depth when more than one person is involved and evaluation has more objectivity. Along with objectivity, collaborative evaluation promotes cooperation and shared responsibility and exposes the client to the ideas, help, and critical appraisal of several persons.

The use of measurable criteria for evaluation of nursing actions provides predictability to the nursing action and reliability to the evaluation. When the criteria for performance are stated in behavioral terms, evaluation is relatively simple. Criteria that are stated in behavioral terms describe the desired outcome of the nursing action, the conditions under which the desired outcome will occur, and the acceptable performance.[13] A number of persons can recognize the desired behavior, thereby providing objectivity to the evaluation, when it is stated in behavioral terms. The more measurable and objective the criteria, the more reliable the evaluation will be; and the more clearly the criteria are stated in behavioral terms, the more probable it is that the nurse will be able to evaluate the nursing action.

Results from the evaluation determine whether the nursing action met the goal, if it needs revision, if it can be repeated, or if another action needs to be considered. If the desired effect is achieved, the intervention has pre-

---

[13]Mager, Robert F.: Preparing instructional objectives, Belmont, 1962, Fearon Publishers, p. 52.

dictability and can be repeated. If the intervention met the immediate goal, it is recorded and remembered for future reference, in case the client has the same need again. Some interventions become part of the individual client's nursing care plan and are utilized repeatedly for the desired effect. These interventions need to be shared with the other members of the health team to provide continuity of care. Some interventions do not achieve the desired effect and are discarded. Again these actions need to be conveyed to the team so that time and energy will not be wasted and the client will not be inconvenienced by others repeating the same useless actions.

In the process of evaluating an intervention, reassessment and another cycle of the nursing process may become necessary. For instance, when medication is given to a client for pain relief, the nurse not only determines if the pain is relieved but if there are any untoward effects from the medication; undesired effects as well as desired effects are determined. If the intervention did not provide the desired effect, the nurse considers other interventions, their consequences, probabilities, value, and risk to determine what to do next. If the intervention provides the desired effect, the nurse evaluates the situation for any other problems. If the nursing intervention provides the desired effect but was expensive of time, energy, and materials, then another alternative with the same positive predictable result might be considered for the future.

Evaluation not only helps determine satisfactory accomplishment of a desired goal or a need for another approach but the need for a change in the criteria. This is especially true of short-term goals. For example, suppose the nursing criterion read, "To prevent pulmonary congestion, urinary congestion, and phlebothrombosis the client will be ambulated for 10 minutes every 4 hours." This statement is particularly useful for the early postoperative period; but after several days it is not necessary for the client to ambulate so restrictively, since he more than likely will be up frequently for long periods of time. The conditions of the criterion need to be changed to meet the changing needs of the client.

Evaluation extracted from feedback on the nursing action is the phase of the decision-making nursing process that determines the validity of the nursing action. It tells the nurse if the action accomplished what it was designed to do. It is an essential part of the nursing process.

SUMMARY

The purpose of this chapter has been to present the nursing process as a decision-making process. The central theme of this chapter is that the process by which the nurse identifies, plans, and implements nursing care is a decision-making process that consists of four phases: (1) assessment, (2) problem identification, (3) formulation of a plan, and (4) planning for evaluation. It is a nursing care process that has multiple feedback mechanisms to ensure evaluation, revision, and flexibility. It is a process that, if utilized consistently, guarantees a systematic, individualized approach to the delivery of nursing care.

This chapter lays the groundwork for the subsequent chapters. Chapter Two presents a theoretical model for the provision of a holistic approach to planning nursing care. Chapter Three presents the concept of assessment and takes the reader through the process of assessing nursing situations. Chapter Four outlines the decision-making process. Chapter Five completes the process by presenting an investigation of the purpose, content, and use of the nursing care plan as a means of activating the nursing decision-making process.

Suggested readings

Bross, L. D. J.: Design for decision, New York, 1953, The Macmillan Company.

Collins, Rosella D.: Problem solving, a tool for patients, too, Amer. J. Nurs. **68**(7):1483-85, 1968.

Douglas, Laura Mae, and Bevis, Em Olivia: Team leadership in action, St. Louis, 1970, The C. V. Mosby Co., pp. 9-22.

Francis, Gloria M.: This thing called problem solving, J. Nurs. Educ. **6**:27-30, 1967.

Kerlinger, Fred N.: Foundations of behavioral research, New York, 1965, Holt, Rinehart & Winston, Inc.

MacDonald, Frederick J.: Educational psychology, Belmont, 1965, Wadsworth Publishing Co., Inc., pp. 59-61.

Schweer, Mildred E., and Gardella, Frances A.: Planning, orienting and preparing for a new kind of nurse leadership, Nurs. Outlook **18**(5):42-46, 1970.

Straus, David, and others: Tools for change, ed. 2, San Francisco, 1971, Interaction Associates, Inc.

Wiedenbach, Ernestine: The helping art of nursing, Amer. J. Nurs. **63**(11):54-57, 1963.

Chapter

A THEORETICAL MODEL FOR PLANNING HOLISTIC NURSING CARE

The invisible shield of caring is a weapon from the sky against being dead.

Source unknown

OVERVIEW

Systematic planning of nursing care is a high-priority concern as nurses seek more efficient ways to provide quality care. Of equal concern to nurses is the manner in which the care is planned. For instance, even if the nurse knows the process, is there any particular approach that has a higher probability of success over any other? Is there an approach that increases the quality of care, that is, increases the quality of the interpersonal action? Is there an approach that effectively provides a humanistic means of meeting the client's needs? For no matter how knowledgeable nurses are about the process of planning care, unless they are able to implement it in some way that is satisfying to both the nurse and the client, the process is useless. This chapter presents an existentialist approach for the planning of holistic care. With this approach the nurse:

1. Recognizes the behavior of the client as an outward sign of his inner experience
2. Believes that until the client discloses his inner intent, an interpretation of his behavior is only guesswork
3. Believes that the client is free to disclose or not to disclose his intents depending on the amount of trust developed between the client and the nurse
4. Believes that the client has the right to be part of planning his own care

The existential approach to planning care is presented as a framework for the process of developing that care. It sets the style and the mode by which the process is carried out. In addition, the concepts of holism, high-level wellness, homeostasis, and stress are discussed and developed into a theoretical model for the assessment and identification of nursing problems.

EXISTENTIALISM AND HUMANISM

The disciplines of existential psychology and humanistic psychology seek to answer the questions: What are the possibilities of man? From these possibilities what is an optimum state for man, and under what conditions is this state most likely to be reached?[1] These disciplines strive to maximize the individuality of man and his full-flowering growth by seeking ways of maximizing or increasing the *odds* for maximization of his potential.

Humanism is a way of life, an attitude or conviction that emphasizes mutual respect and recognizes human interdependence. The humanistic approach aims at the development of the highest potential of the individual.[2]

Existential psychology emphasizes the dimension of will and decision. Clients do not "happen" to make decisions by default, fatigue, or because of a need for approval. Nor are decisions made for them. The existential approach puts decisions and will into the center of things; it operates on the premise that "in the revealing and exploring of [the] determinative forces in the patient's life, the patient is orienting himself in some particular way to the data and thus is engaged in some choice, no matter how seemingly insignificant; is experiencing some freedom, no matter how subtle."[3]

Health care involves the diagnosis and analysis of the client's difficulties, the cautious interpretation and explanation to the client of his difficulties, and a reeducative phase. An interaction between the client and the clinician that involves the client in the exploring, analyzing, and understanding of the difficulties promotes a concomitant sense of responsibility by the client to the outcome. It acknowledges his rights and freedom as an individual. To create this kind of climate a humanistic approach is needed. Planning nursing care that is aimed at helping the individual reach his highest potential and that encourages him to develop problem-solving skills requires a nurse who has learned to behave in ways that can achieve these two essential goals.

Over the years health care professionals have conceptualized man as a machine, as an organism, as a communicative system, as a computer—and have fallen short of perceiving his wholeness and uniqueness as a human being.

Nurses can choose either (1) to treat clients as objects for cure and to plan

---

[1] Jourard, Sidney M.: Disclosing man to himself, Princeton, 1968, D. Van Nostrand Co., Inc., p. 3.

[2] Fact sheet, American Humanist Association, San Francisco, 1970, Humanist House.

[3] May, Rollo: Existential psychology, Copyright 1960, Random House, Inc., pp. 43-44.

care that does things for and to the client but that seems to achieve only part of the nursing goals; or (2) to try an approach that encourages the individual to meet his potential. There are some concepts that form the theoretical basis for a humanistic existential nursing approach and are therefore basic to nursing care. They are as follows:

1. Man is free to make decisions that affect him.
2. Man is free to be involved in his own plan of care.

These two concepts have implications for nursing care, since they indicate that the nursing role is one of assistance. Nurses help clients as they seek ways to maximize their growth and discover the intrinsic and environmental conditions that make self-actualization possible. As the nurse plans care, consideration of the client as a *participating member* of the health team becomes evident. Not only is he encouraged to become involved but he is also viewed as a major part of the decision-making process, if not *the* major decision maker. Respect is given to the client regardless of a difference in goals. The nurse listens, sorts, and reinforces any attempts the client initiates as he makes decisions that move him toward optimal health. Nursing goals are separated from client goals and each is evaluated in light of its chances for goal attainment.

Understanding human behavior

To understand the essence of anything two things are necessary. If the subject is an inanimate object, such as a star or a stone, or is an animate object, such as a bacterium, the problem of discovery depends on making contact with the object and then of devising some means of unfolding its mysteries. Natural scientists have shown incredible sophistication in this task. They have devised gadgets that reveal amazing phenomena about things, objects, and processes in the world. To gain knowledge and understand man is a different task. Existentialists have stated that man is a being who is evolving, who is not fixed in time or space, who chooses his way of life and the way he relates to others. Each man therefore is free to relate, to move, to exist in a different way. He has the option of showing his inner self. If he chooses to show himself, he will freely be himself. His behavior, which is an outward expression of his inner experience, demonstrates his goals and intentions. But the observer can only guess at the meaning of his behavior, since the key to understanding it lies with the behaver. People will disclose the meaning of their behavior, their goals, and their intent only with the help of those they trust. Without trust a person will hide or misrepresent his inner experiences in hopes of getting the observer to misconstrue the visible behavior. This does not imply that the individual always knows why he behaves as he does; it simply means he will not attempt to discover or reveal the meaning of his behavior if he does not trust the other person.

According to Jourard there are two kinds of interpersonal encounters—

those that mystify and those that reveal.[4] In mystifying encounters one individual manipulates the other. For example:

> A young man hospitalized with a severe chronic lung infection finds himself in isolation. Fearful of what is happening to him but not wanting others to know of his fears, the young man acts indifferent and even jovial at times. At the same time he is constantly calling for something. He requests assistance with his daily hygiene, with eating, and with many other activities that he could handle himself.

Without knowledge of the boy's fears, his behavior is only a string of responses that could mean anything. To understand his actions the nurse must know what his actions mean to him. His behavior is therefore mystifying.

On the other hand, in encounters that reveal, each person experiences the other as a person. It does not matter whether there is verbal or nonverbal exchange. The aim is to show oneself honestly. The threat that motivates people to conceal their intentions and experiences in manipulative encounters is absent. The objective that makes the behavior of each understood by the other is fully realized. Trust is the natural outcome of such an encounter.

Gaining knowledge of another in encounters that are revealing demands a humanistic approach; an approach that encourages a free exchange of thoughts and feelings. Nurse-client relationships are humanistic, when the nurse seeks to know the client by taking steps to find out who and how he is. Some of these steps are as follows:

1. Creating a relationship in which the client discloses the meaning of his behavior
2. Identifying and understanding the factors that create symptoms or behaviors
3. Encouraging the client to disclose his inner experiences
4. Creating a relationship in which the client is exposed and encouraged to relate to a nurse who is warm, concerned, and responsive

Value of a humanistic approach to the client

A client who is cared for by a nurse utilizing the humanistic approach is more than comfortable. He knows what is being done for him because he is involved in his plan of care; he feels his nurse knows him as a unique person because the nurse took the trouble to learn about him; he feels free to ask for help when he wants it because he has been encouraged to do so. And his nurse is interested enough in him to have sampled his personal and private world.

---

[4] Jourard: Disclosing man to himself, pp. 19-21.

Nurses who are humanistic have the ability to see what is common to all mankind, yet to differentiate what is unique to each individual. They know that hope, purpose, meaning, and direction promote wellness; that one's attitudes toward life and self are factors that affect one's health. One of the events that inspires hope and purpose in people is the conviction that someone cares. The quality then of the nurse-client relationship is a major factor in the client's recovery.

Factors that affect the humanistic relationship

Many factors affect the nurse's ability to create a humanistic relationship, such as (1) the setting (environment), (2) the characteristics of the nurse and the client, (3) the willingness of the nurse to get involved in a personal way, and (4) the nurse's ability to remain professional, that is, to provide guidance while creating a humanistic relationship.

Creating a therapeutic environment

Nurses have the major responsibility for creating an environment that is conducive to problem solving and the resolution of conflicts. The physical and the interpersonal environments greatly affect the client's progress.

The physical environment of the acute hospital, the outpatient clinic, or the rehabilitation unit needs to simulate the real world. Rooms that are colorful, attractive, and comfortable enhance the client's feelings of security and his sense of well-being. Policies, schedules, and procedures that meet the client's needs, the staff's needs, and the agency's protocol facilitate client progress. As the nurse considers and plans for environmental change, the goals and the philosophy of the agency need to be considered. Inclusion of meaningful people and objects in the client's environment promotes a sense of security and well-being. Visiting hours that are flexible (allowing relatives and friends the opportunity to visit at convenient times) and having personal belongings close at hand provide the kind of environment that reduces the feeling of strangeness and fear. Personal belongings, such as pictures of loved ones and food from home, decrease the sense of isolation and change, the strangeness and threat of hospitalization.

Of major concern in the development of a therapeutic environment is the inclusion of the client in decisions that concern and affect him. When the client helps make the decision, he is involved in the nursing care planning and is thus committed to the decision and is more likely willing to take an active part in achieving a state of high-level wellness.

Interpersonal environment

The interpersonal environment is a crucial part of the humanistic relationship. Free and open communication is essential. The creation of a safe environment that is open and free is only possible if nurses have an awareness of their own attitudes, prejudices, and values. Often nurses are expected to be nonjudgmental. Such a state is not possible. All humans make judgments, since each individual has his own unique value system. If it is in opposition or in conflict with the client's value system, the nurse can then openly acknowledge the difference and deal with it. Rather than attempt to do the impossible, that is, be nonjudgmental, nurses need to accept their prejudices and biases. To accept the client means that the nurse acknowledges his difference and accepts him for what he is and what he believes. Acceptance of another does not mean acceptance of the other's values and beliefs. The ability to accept the client not only allows for open and free communication, but creates a trusting relationship, a vital component of a therapeutic relationship.

Characteristics of nurse and client

The nurse who plans and carries out humanistic nursing care is an individual who has the expertise to assist the client as he seeks optimal well-being. The nurse's preparation and experience enable her to assess situations, to identify and set priorities, and to propose and carry out nursing actions. Nurses bring with them a background in the natural and behavioral sciences and the humanities, which allows them not only to understand the nature of human beings and to respect the dignity and uniqueness of each individual but also to plan care accordingly. Nurses prepared in these areas are able to share their knowledge and expertise with other nurses and health workers acting to develop the planning skills of others. Since the major goal for all nurses is the promotion of health and the prevention of illness, nurses encourage the public to develop habits of health care; they counsel, teach, and model good health practices in order to promote behavioral change in others. Because nurses are required by the nature of their functions to move with the changing times, they are inquisitive, innovative, and motivated toward increasing their knowledge and skills; nurses do not merely seek solutions but are willing to propose, initiate, and create innovative answers. Most of all, nurses who are humanistic are caring, sensitive persons who give much of themselves as they become involved in providing care. In essense, they are persons who (1) care, (2) comfort, (3) contribute, and (4) consult.

Clients come from many different ethnic, cultural groups, from different economic and geographic groups, and from different social interaction groups. The common component of all clients is their need for help to prevent disease and to maintain or reach optimal health. The individual seeking help may be anywhere on the spectrum of health from deviation to deprivation. The individual may be actively responding to his predicament or passively accepting his state. His level of dependency may be anywhere from total dependence to complete independence, depending on many factors. He may be aware of a problem or he may be totally unaware of a health need, and he may be unaware of his own contribution to the health problem. Often nurses intervene to prevent potential problems that the individual cannot recognize. In all instances nurses seek not only to interact with the identified client, but to be critically tuned in to the needs and level of health of other members of the family. The nurse is also concerned about the factors in the community that affect the client.

Nurses' individual characteristics and clients' individual characteristics, with such a wide variety and differentiation, demand that nurses assess, critically analyze, and evaluate each situation in order to create a humanistic relationship.

Humanism and professionalism

If the aim of humanistic approach is to develop man's optimal potential, then, unlike other approaches, it is not only concerned with the factors that affect man's experience and action but is also concerned with liberating the individual from the impact of these factors so that he can pursue his freedom and growth. Nurses who enter into a humanistic relationship by revealing themselves as real people give their clients a chance to pursue the path to freedom and health in two ways. One way is by modeling realness, humanness, and by creating a climate for free interaction. The other way is by the gentle but firm guidance the nurse provides for the client as he is led toward the discovery of the factors that affect his life, and ways and means by which he can liberate or free himself from these factors. The professional character of the relationship lies in the nurse's ability to give of self while providing direction for the client.

HOLISTIC THEORY

Man not only responds as an individual in a unique manner but also as a total organism. Man is a whole consisting of millions of parts. These parts are in the form of cells of many kinds, and the cells are smaller wholes of indefinite complexity. All the parts are coordinated and function with the most complete collaboration in support of each other and the whole organism. All the various activities of the several parts and organs seem directed to central ends; there is thus cooperation and unified action of the organism as a whole instead of the separate mechanical activities of the parts. Mind and body are not separate entities, nor does the mind consist of independent faculties or elements separate from body organs and processes. What happens in one part affects the whole.[5]

Wholeness implies that the individual is seeking his optimal potential as a

---

[5]Smuts, J. C.: Holism and evolution, New York, 1926, The Macmillan Company, pp. 85-117.

complete well-integrated whole. He strives to be alert, to grow, to develop, and to perform the acts of daily living with interest, enjoyment, and satisfaction. To cope constructively with the stresses of life, to face reality, and to relate to other people, family, and community in a satisfying and contributory manner, demonstrate optimum health. Health problems arise when (1) there is an imbalance among the components of the whole (2) a component of the whole disrupts the whole, or (3) there is a misinterpretation of the situation.

Health problems that arise from an imbalance among the components of the whole may be caused by a breakdown in the interrelatedness of the various parts or from a weakening of one of the components of the whole. An example would be the inability of the regulatory mechanisms of the body to maintain balance, such as the acid-base regulatory mechanisms. If the pH of the body, which indicates the acidity or the alkalinity, becomes too acidic or too alkaline, serious problems result. Normally, various buffering systems regulate chemical shifts and keep the pH within a range that is compatible with life. But if these buffers, for one reason or another, are unable to keep the body's acid-base balance within these limits, the whole body responds. The body's chemical and physiological processes are affected, often causing the person to become dehydrated, hallucinatory, and delusional. If unattended the person may lapse into a coma and eventually die.

Health problems also occur when one of the components of the whole disrupts the whole. These problems include not only the effects to the disrupted part but the disruptive effect to the whole body. For instance, an acute inflamed appendix has a local and a systemic effect; a herniated lumbar disk creates local pain and spasm, which in turn, limits the person's motor activity, which in turn, may affect the person's job performance. Alcoholism not only disrupts the liver, brain, and eventually the whole central nervous system but also disrupts the individual's relationships with his family, his job, and other persons. Health problems can arise from a person's response to the disruption he is experiencing. The parent who is grieving over the death of a child often experiences a lack of motivation and has little interest in the acts of daily living. He cannot sleep, is anorexic, unkempt, and withdrawn. He is responding to his loss in a holistic manner; psychologically, physically, and socially he is reacting to the loss of a loved one. Sometimes the response to a health problem is the result of the individual's interpretation of the problem. The person with coronary heart disease who views himself as a "cardiac cripple" could disrupt a family and do unnecessary damage to himself. Believing that he should not exert himself because of his heart problem, he may avoid exercise, demand that the family members do everything for him, and as a result be eliminating a valuable part of his rehabilitation and be placing unrealistic expectations on the family.

Much like the individual, the family is a whole that is affected by what happens to its parts; the health problems of the members can affect the family's pattern of living, its role assignments, and its integrity. Some members may be supportive, whereas others are critical of a person as demanding as the man with the cardiac problem described above. If the family members are supportive, the family unity or wholeness remains intact. But if the members split, with some supportive and others critical, then the unity of the family is threatened, often necessitating outside help. The same holistic concept is true of communities. The health problems of a community are the symptoms of a larger, more complex community problem. Drug abuse, venereal disease, malnutrition, and a rising incidence of suicide are all symptoms of pathological conditions in the community. Many communities seek to correct these problems, as they should, but it remains essential that the whole social problem be considered also. Research and study of the community's social stratification and the degree of integration, the stresses, the employment-unemployment ratio and job opportunities, the available community resources, and the political structure are needed if its health problems are to be corrected. Unless the factors that create the symptoms are discovered and corrected, no permanent solution to the problem is possible. The whole community structure must be considered when attempting to handle any health problem, for no part of the whole functions without its impact on the other parts and on the whole.

Interdependent nature of health problems

Health problems may precipitate or potentiate other problems. The potential problems of lung congestion, skin breakdown, stasis of urine, bowel obstruction, and personality deterioration are all possible when an elderly individual suffers a severe cerebral vascular accident and is bedridden and paralyzed. Anxiety and conflict over job performance can precipitate coping behaviors that create either peptic ulcers, migraine headaches, or acute anxiety reactions. Man cannot be a physical or an emotional health problem alone, for he reacts to his world as a whole with the many parts of the whole responding as a whole to the environment.

Creative impulse of holism

A deteriorating or malfunctioning part does not negate the concept of wholeness. Wholeness is realized by the development of the corresponding parts to again create a whole; by maximizing the healthy parts, keeping in mind the impact of the deteriorating condition on the whole, the body compensates to create wholeness. Because organization is built into the system and the integrity of the organism is not permitted to be lost by the deterioration of a part, the total being acts as one to reorganize itself into a new whole.

Goals of nursing care

"Health is a state of complete physical, mental, and social well-being, and not merely the absence of disease and infirmity."[6] This particular definition is part of the preamble to the Constitution of the World Health Organization. Health obviously means more than the absence of illness. It includes well-being within the family and the community. It certainly means that the environment needs to be one that encourages the individual to live life to the very fullest.

H. L. Dunn's concept of wellness states:

> High-level wellness for the individual is defined as an integrated method of functioning which is oriented toward maximizing the potential which the individual is capable of. It requires that the individual maintain a continuum of balance and purposeful direction within the environment where he is functioning.[7]

Dunn's concept of wellness embodies the individual's, the family's, and the community's quest for optimum health and not just the fighting of disease, disability, and social breakdown. It encompasses the preventive aspects of health care and accounts for the individuality of each man, family, and community. It also engulfs the concept of holism. He speaks of "integrated method of functioning" in the sense of interrelatedness of the total individual and of maximizing as a means of maintaining completeness. Existentially, Dunn's definition also implies a "becoming," since his use of the word maximizing has a dynamic meaning, not a static one. The definition does not imply there is an optimum level of wellness, but rather that wellness is the direction toward an ever higher potential.

Beeson describes health as "a ceaseless struggle between a basically hostile environment and a series of defenses we are endowed with . . . . The homeostatic balance of forces is our goal and this may be accomplished by decreasing the thrust of the environment or by raising the capacity of the host to defend itself."[8] Beeson's definition of health emphasizes the individual's need to adapt to a constantly changing environment to remain healthy. Homeostasis as explained by Cannon is the coordinated physiological processes that maintain most of the steady state of the organism.[9] It involves the maintenance of cellular activity within well-defined limits. This maintenance depends on a variety of factors. The supply of substances required by the cells must be available in sufficient quantity. They must include energy,

---

[6]World Health Organization, Constitution of the World Health Organization, Chronicle of the World Health Organization 1(1-2):29-43,1947.
[7]Dunn, Halbert L.: High-level wellness, Virginia, 1961, R. W. Beatty, Ltd., pp. 4-7.
[8]Beeson, Gerald: The health-illness spectrum, Amer. J. Public Health 57:1904, 1967.
[9]Cannon, Walter B.: The wisdom of the body, New York, 1939, W. W. Norton & Company, Inc., p. 24.

tissue-building substances, electrolytes, and regulators not already present in the body. The intake, storage, and elimination of excesses are regulated within very definite limits and the condition of the external environment must be within the limits to which man can adapt.

Beeson's definition of health and Cannon's concept of homeostasis both support and amplify Dunn's concept of high-level wellness. Homeostasis in this sense is a state of balance in which energy forces within the body interact and interrelate to act against or with the forces of the environment.

STRESS RESPONSE

If a state of high-level wellness requires homeostatic balance between man and his environment, then any force, either from the environment or from within man that threatens that balance, precipitates a state of disequilibrium or "illness." After years of study of the "syndrome of just being sick," Hans Selye coined the word "stress" to describe "the sum of all the nonspecific effects of factors that can act upon the body."[10] In 1936 Selye first defined stress as "the rate at which we live at any moment. All living things are constantly under stress and anything pleasant or unpleasant, that speeds up the intensity of life causes a temporary increase in stress."[11] Stress does not, according to Selye, consist merely of damage but also of adaptation to damage. Stress can be scientifically analyzed and objectively appraised by certain characteristic changes in the structural and chemical composition of the body. Selye named the agent that precipitates stress the "stressor."[12]

Later, George Engel defined stress as "any influence, whether it arises from the internal environment or the external environment, which interferes with the satisfaction of basic needs or which threatens to disturb the stable equilibrium."[13] Selye's stress syndrome focuses on the physiological responses and adaptations of the human body to stressors, whether internal or external. Stress to Selye is the *effect*, the body's response to factors that act on man, whereas stress as defined by Engel is the *cause* of the response—the factor that threatens the homeostasis of the body. To avoid confusion, the concept of stress as used in this presentation refers to those environmental, interpersonal, and intrapersonal factors that act on man to disturb his

---

[10]Selye, Hans: The stress of life, copyright 1956, McGraw-Hill Book Company, p. 42. Used with permission of McGraw-Hill Book Company.
[11]Selye, Hans: The stress syndrome, Amer. J. Nurs. **65**:97-99, 1965, Copyright American Journal of Nursing Company.
[12]Selye: The stress of life, p. 64.
[13]Engle, George: Homeostasis, behavioral adjustment and the concept of health and disease. In Grinker, Roy R., editor: Mid-century psychiatry, Springfield, Ill., 1953, Charles C Thomas, Publisher, p. 51.

homeostasis. And those processes or behaviors that occur as a result of the stress will be referred to as the *response* to stress.

To develop a state of high-level wellness the individual or the family needs to adjust to constant change. Since life is largely a process of adaptation to the circumstances in which we live and the secret of health lies in successful adjustment to these circumstances, the ability to cope is paramount for survival. Successful coping creates homeostasis and homeostasis provides man with an avenue for pursuing high-level wellness.

Stress and anxiety

Stress produces anxiety, leading to an adaptive response that may or may not be effective. Stress may be external in origin, such as an invasion by bacteria or from the pressures of the social system. It may be internal in origin and arise from the individual's interpretation of a situation as threatening or from an internal response to a physiological change, such as a fluid and electrolyte imbalance. Stress elicits a protective response that acts to satisfy needs, avoid danger, or achieve a goal. This response is holistic in that there are physiological and psychological components that mobilize the body for adaptation.

Anxiety is a universal experience shared by all humans. It is subjectively experienced as an uncomfortable feeling of apprehension. Such feelings as muscle tension, nausea, and dread are accompanied by an increase in the pulse and respiratory rate, tremor, and sometimes diarrhea. A sense of uncertainty and helplessness is often present. The degree of anxiety determines the individual's ability to function. Mild anxiety is experienced as a vague discomfort, an uncertainty or excitement. As the anxiety increases the response may progress to create a hyperactive sympathetic nervous system and a situation in which the individual cannot function. High levels of anxiety decrease the individual's perceptual field; he sees and hears very little. His perceptual field narrows, since he can only concentrate on one thing at a time. High levels of anxiety can lead to psychotic behavior. When anxiety becomes unbearable, panic and terror result. Psychotic behavior is both the expression of the anxiety and the individual's attempt to cope with it.

Anxiety is not always destructive. Anxiety serves as a danger signal that mobilizes the individual toward constructive activity. For example, a mild level of anxiety is necessary to motivate the individual to seek safety in a threatening situation or to explore new ways to manage in an ever-changing world. Anxiety serves as a stimulus to growth and learning. In fact, it is questionable whether the human race would have survived without this universal phenomenon. Therefore it is important for man to maintain a level of anxiety that encourages constructive activity. A healthy person and a healthy society are ones in which there is a level of anxiety that maintains vitality and promotes growth.

STRESS-RESPONSE MODEL

Planning nursing care that is individualized, that promotes high-level wellness, and that is holistic is not only needed but possible. One way to deal with man and his response to stress in an ever-changing world is to utilize a systems approach. As Banathy states in his preface to *Instructional Systems,* "in the systems approach we have a methodology the use of which empowers us to explore and manage complex entities. In fact, we may have here something by which we cannot only cope with our environment but also be able to shape and master it and make change work for us."[14] With the systems approach the organization of the whole is considered by determining how the parts interact to make the whole. Systems theory is concerned with purpose, process, and content. Purpose gives direction to the system and process determines the means by which the system accomplishes the purpose. The nature of the process suggests the component parts ot the content of the system.

The author proposes a stress-response systems model as a means of organizing data to create a holistic approach to planning nursing care. The stress-response model is a conceptual organization of ideas, theories, and concepts. It is designed to help the nurse develop a frame of reference whereby the interrelatedness of man and his universe can be understood. The model proposes a matrix of ideas that symbolize man and his environment in their wholeness. It rests on the basic premises that have been discussed so far, which are as follows:

1. Man is a system with purpose, process, and content.
2. Man's purpose is self-actualized high-level wellness.
3. Man's processes are those that enable and promote the purpose of high-level wellness.
4. Man's content is all the factors that make up the processes.
5. Man is homeostatic in nature.

Man's life processes maintain optimum health by their constant balancing effect. They neutralize, compensate, and interact to the internal and external forces that tend to create an imbalance. Man is an individual with coping mechanisms that respond to the stresses of life to maintain a homeostatic balance.

The most important concept of the stress-response model is its wholeness. The model depicts man as a unified whole having his own distinctive characteristics that cannot be perceived by looking at the parts. However, a summation of the parts does not add up to a whole man. Man as a whole interacts with the whole environment. Changes taking place in man and in the environment are holistic. Pattern and organization give individuality to each

---

[14]Banathy, Bela H.: Instructional systems, Belmont, 1968, Fearon Publishers, pp. iii-iv.

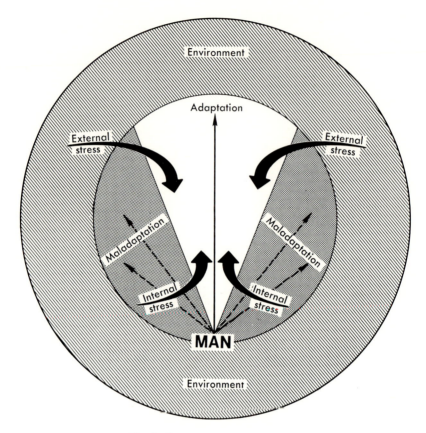

Fig. 3. Stress-response model.

man and alterations in the organization or pattern are continuous. Man as conceptualized by the model evolves in totality. Fig. 3 is a representation of the stress-response model. It demonstrates man's struggle to balance the inner forces and tensions with the environmental forces as he strives to reach his potential. The solid arrow in the middle represents the dynamic forces that control the energy created by the interaction. The two black lines on either side of the arrow outline the nonshaded area that is labeled adaptation and designates the adaptive limits of this dynamic process. When the compensatory mechanisms of man are unable to maintain homeostasis, that is, maintain a state of balance within man and between man and the environment, then the arrow moves either to one side or the other. If the arrow dips too far either way, it moves out of the nonshaded area and swings into areas of deviation from the normal—into areas of maladaptation. Man cannot reach his optimal potential when he is too far outside the limits of adaptation. The extremes of the spectrum result in deprivation (insufficiencies) or distortion (excesses). In either case the individual is out of balance; he is functioning in a maladaptive manner. For example, proliferation of cell growth, hyper-thyroidism, and manic behavior, to name a few, are conditions that are in excess. They are distortions of the normal. Diabetes, anemia, and dehydration are conditions that are the result of insufficiencies. They are deprivations. Man seeks to cope with his stresses by remaining close to the center of the model to stay within the adaptive range. Man's striving to acquire maximum growth in wholeness is demonstrated by the arrow, which reaches its greatest height at the center.

The stress-response model can be utilized by the nurse to identify client or family needs or problems and to determine the appropriate nursing intervention. By identifying the stress and the coping response, the nurse can determine the nursing need and act accordingly.[15]

Nursing interventions and the stress-response model

Nursing is a process that promotes health, prevents illness, and helps man develop behaviors for handling stress. Nursing action is directed toward the goal of helping the individual cope effectively with his environment. Over a hundred years ago Florence Nightingale described nursing as a process that "puts the patient in the best condition for nature to act upon him."[16] But with the rapid advances in medical technology, the knowledge explosion, and the expansion of health facilities, it has become necessary to describe nursing behaviors in a more up-to-date manner. Martha Rogers describes nursing as the ability to "assist man in moving as far as possible in the direction of maximum health."[17] Em Olivia Bevis states, "Nursing is a process; its purpose is to promote optimum health through protective, nurtrative[18] and generative activities. These activities are carried out within the intrapersonal, interpersonal and community systems. Nursing's protective, nurtrative and generative activities are derived from a unique synthesis of theories combined into nursing hypotheses which are validated or refuted in practice."[19]

If nursing is concerned with assisting the individual toward high-level wellness, then three types of nursing behaviors are possible: supportive, generative, and protective. Underlying these three nursing interventions, the

---

[15]Refer to Chapter Three for an example of how to use the stress-response model to determine nursing needs.

[16]Nightingale, Florence: Notes on nursing, London, 1859, Harris & Sons, p. 75.

[17]Rogers, Martha: Educational revolution in nursing, New York, 1967, The Macmillan Company, p. 23.

[18]A coined word.

[19]Bevis, Em Olivia: Curriculum building in nursing: a process, St. Louis, The C. V. Mosby Co. (To be published in 1973.)

nurse must base her actions on the following premises:
1. Man has the right to decide his destiny and to be involved in decisions that affect him.
2. Nursing intervention is designed to *assist* the individual to meet his own individual needs or to solve his individual problems.
3. The ultimate goal of all nursing interventions is to assist the individual to the point where he can assume responsibility for his own actions.

Supportive nursing actions. Nursing measures that provide comfort, treatment, and promote restoration are supportive nursing actions. They help the individual cope more effectively with stress. They augment and complement the individual's present adaptive coping behaviors to arrest the health problem and prevent further problems. By maximizing the individual's strengths and providing encouragement, relief, and guidance, the individual is able to successfully regain his health.

> A middle-aged executive is troubled by insomnia, hypertension, and stomach pains. He is overweight and has recently been diagnosed to have ulcers. He is concerned about his obesity and wishes to lose weight. His physician refers him to the industrial nurse where he works for health guidance. The nurse helps him plan meals that fit his prescribed diet, encourages his interest and his attempts to exercise, praises his weight loss, and encourages the expression of his feelings and concerns. In a while he is sleeping better, has lost a little weight, and has a considerably lower blood pressure.

The nurse in this example utilized the gentleman's interest and concern by involving him in his plan of care and built his therapy around his desire to change. She encouraged him, praised him, and helped him regain health by building on his strengths; she helped him cope with his health problem as she gave him the guidance and support he needed.

Supportive nursing actions provide the client with comfort; when he is in pain, is too hot or too cold, or is just miserable, the nurse intervenes to relieve the pain, to provide warmth or coolness, and to do what is necessary to alleviate the misery. Supportive nursing measures provide dignity for the dying and offer assistance to the grieving. These actions demonstrate that the nurse cares. When the nurse makes a bed, dresses a wound, or gives an enema, she is offering comfort, promoting restoration, and providing treatment.

Generative nursing actions. Measures that are innovative, rehabilitative, and productive are generative nursing actions. They are those nursing measures that help the individual develop new or different approaches for coping with stress. Because the client's present coping behaviors are too limited to handle the health problem or his usual methods are ineffective and he is anxious for resolution, he is willing to try something different. The mother of a teenager who is involved in drug abuse seeks help when she finds that her daughter and she have reached an impasse and can no longer communicate. The nurse encourages them to express their feelings, to listen to one another, and to accept each other's differences. By learning new or better skills for communicating, the mother and her daughter can then tackle the drug abuse problem.

Generative nursing actions are particularly useful for those individuals struggling with a new role, a change in role, or an identity crisis. A middle-aged man who suffered a coronary infarct was bathed, fed, and waited on early in his hospitalization to reduce the work load of his heart. These nursing measures were supportive, since they helped maintain the vital function of his heart. After an extended period of hospitalization, generative nursing actions were used to prepare him for return to his home. Limited activity and diet restrictions were discussed with him and plans were made that incorporated these restrictions into his home life. Follow-up by a Community Health Nurse provided him with support as he adjusted to his new modified role. As time passed, the nurse offered suggestions and introduced innovative ideas and possibilities, as she helped him develop ways to handle his modified role.

Generative nursing actions are extremely helpful in assisting those who are trying to establish an identity. A 19-year-old boy struggling with a dependence-independence conflict was referred to an outpatient clinic for group therapy. In the past two years he had run away from home four times, had dropped out of school, and had had frequent episodes of behavioral swings from maniac to depressive. Nursing actions for this boy included helping him develop new ways to handle his anxiety and conflicts. By learning to identify and express his feelings, by examining his behavior and learning to identify and look at the consequences of his acts, he was able to reduce his anxiety and cope with his conflicts. Although he is still in therapy, he has less frequent mood swings and is better able to verbalize his concerns and communicate his feelings to others, and he does not run away from home any more.

Generative nursing measures are rehabilitative also. From the time the health problem becomes evident until the individual has resolved the problem he needs assistance in dealing with the many changes inherent in the situation. The nurse explores, considers, and designs ways and means of helping the client meet his needs and reestablish himself as a productive member of society.

Protective nursing actions. Nursing measures that promote health and prevent disease are protective nursing actions. They are measures that improve or correct situations. For instance, let us consider the newborn infant who is choking on mucous. Since the infant is born with an active gag reflex but without an expulsive cough reflex, it is necessary for the nurse to intervene to prevent aspiration or asphyxiation. The most effective nurse action would be to turn the infant upside down and pat him gently on the back to drain the mucous from his bronchial tree. Immunizations, health teaching, anticipatory guidance, genetic counseling, and early intervention to prevent complications and sequelae of illness are all examples of protective nursing actions. The school nurse who cleanses the abraded knee of a child prevents infection by providing an environment conducive for healing.

Supportive, generative, and protective nursing actions are not mutually exclusive. They can occur simultaneously or separately. They quite often occur together to provide optimal nursing care.

SUMMARY

The process of planning nursing care that is individualized, holistic, and directed toward maintaining homeostasis toward high-level wellness may be achieved by: (1) utilizing a stress-response model for the identification of nursing problems; (2) systematically making nursing decisions based on an existential philosophy; and (3) evaluating the outcome of nursing decisions utilizing the goal of maximum growth toward optimal functioning.

This chapter has explored humanism as a means of implementing planned nursing care. It has presented the concepts of stress and homeostasis as the basic components of a stress-response model. It is the purpose of the remainder of this book to (1) demonstrate the use of the model for the identification of nursing problems, (2) guide the nurse in the steps of decision-making when planning holistic nursing care, and (3) provide the nurse with a means of communicating the plan of nursing action to others.

Suggested readings

Banathy, Bela H.: Instructional systems, Belmont, 1968, Fearon Publishers.
Bennis, Warren G., Beene, Kenneth D., and Chin, Robert: The planning of change: readings in the applied behavioral sciences, New York, 1962, Holt, Rinehart & Winston, Inc., pp. 202-203.
Brinling, Trudy: Tearing down a wall, Amer. J. Nurs. 71(7):1406-1409, 1971.
Brown, Esther Lucille: Newer dimensions of patient care, New York, 1962, The Russell Sage Foundation.
Dunn, Halbert L.: High-level wellness, Washington, D. C., 1961, R. W. Beatty, Ltd.
Hazzard, Mary Elizabeth: An overview of systems theory, Nurs. Clin. N. Amer. 6(3):385-393, 1971.
Jourard, Sidney M.: The transparent self, Princeton, 1964, D. Van Nostrand Co., Inc.
Langner, Thomas S., and Michael, Stanley T.: Life, stress and mental health, vol. 2., London, 1963, The Free Press of Glencoe.
May, Rollo.: Love and will, New York, 1969, W. W. Norton & Company, Inc.
Rodgers, Carl.: On becoming a person, Boston, 1961, Houghton Mifflin Company.

Ruesch, Jergen: Therapeutic communication, New York, 1961, W. W. Norton & Company, Inc.

Selye, Hans: The stress of life, New York, 1956, McGraw-Hill Book Company, pp. 127, 166, 171, 177.

Shostrom, Everett L.: Man, the manipulator, New York, 1967, Bantam Books, Inc.

Chapter

3

IDENTIFYING NURSING PROBLEMS UTILIZING THE
STRESS-RESPONSE MODEL

A teacher used to start his first class of each term by putting two figures on the blackboard: four and two.

"What's the solution?" he would ask.

A student would call out, "Six." Another would say, "Two." Several would shout the final possibility, "Eight." And the teacher would shake his head. Finally he would say, "All you failed to ask the key question: *What is the problem?* Unless you know what the problem is, you cannot possibly find the answer. Too much time is spent trying to solve the wrong problem—like polishing brass on a sinking ship."

Source unknown

OVERVIEW

Planned individualized nursing care begins with a complete and accurate assessment of the individual's, the family's, or the community's needs. It is predicated upon the fact that each man is a unique individual, each family a unit with distinct characteristics, and each community a system specifically constructed to meet the needs of particular groups of people. Assessment is a continuous process that provides data for planning and modifying nursing care. It begins with the nurse's initial encounter with a nursing situation. By definition, assessment is the process of "analyzing critically and definitively judging the nature, significance, status and merit of a situation."[1] A thorough and complete assessment yields valuable data for the identification of patient, family, or community needs. It also enables the nurse to identify problem areas.

Assessment requires the following tasks:

---

[1] Merriam-Webster, A.: Webster's third new international dictionary, Unabridged, vol. I, Chicago, 1966, William Benton, p. 131.

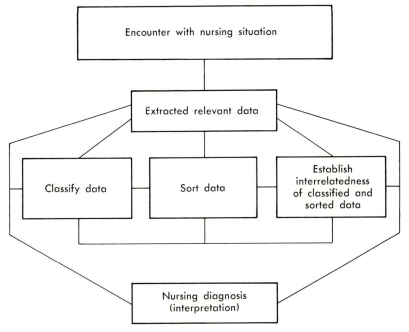

Fig. 4. Process of assessment.

1. Extracting relevant facts and concepts from the situation
2. Classifying and sorting these data into groups that demonstrate relationships
3. Making interpretations of the situation based on the interrelatedness of these groupings

A determination of the individual's, the family's, or the community's health needs begins with data collection. Data collected from many sources are analyzed, classified, and summarized to determine nursing problems and nursing interventions. The process of gathering data is complex and systematic, but is an absolutely vital component to the formulation of a relevant nursing care plan.

This chapter (1) explores the process of assessment, the first phase of the process of planning care; (2) demonstrates the use of the stress-response model in determining nursing problems from the assessment.

PROCESS OF COLLECTING DATA

Data for assessing health needs are obtained from several sources. Interviews, health care records, observations, diagnostic tests, family and friends, and other health professionals are a few of the many sources available for data collection. These data comprise the nursing history. By definition, the nursing history is all the information about the person, family, or the community that has preceded the present health situation; it is all the information that may influence the present or future nursing care needs. Nursing histories indicate the individual's or the family's potentiality and their attitudes toward achieving maximum health status. The nursing history establishes the direction and scope of the nursing care.

Nursing history

   Data from interviews with the client, his friends, or family alert the nurse to the client's

1. Previous experiences with illness and hospitalization and their meaning to the individual
2. Level of knowledge and how he interprets his health problem, diagnosis, and therapeutic regimen
3. Occupational and social roles
4. Educational and intellectual capacity
5. Recreational, religious, and usual health practices
6. Language usage
7. Economic status and employment patterns
8. Level of behavioral growth and development
9. Present and past coping behaviors utilized for handling stress
10. Usual cultural patterns of daily living (This includes food preferences, hygienic and sleep patterns, elimination routines, as well as the interfamily relationships and type of neighborhood living style.)
11. Relationships with others, particularly those others who are "significant" (Who are the "significant" or important people that influence the life and decisions of the client?)

The nursing history is not a replication of the medical or social history, but it will include some medical and social aspects. Because the nursing history is holistic, it will include medical and social information that is pertinent to nursing care. For example, the nurse might note in the medical history that the client had sought help over a year ago for a similar health problem. The record might not tell the nurse why the client sought help, what help was dispensed, how the help was utilized, or if it alleviated the problem. The nursing history includes answers to all these questions and provides the nurse with relevant data to make valid decisions about the nursing care. The content of the nursing history varies according to the type of care sought and the limitations and philosophy of the agency that offers the care.

   Previous experiences with illness or hospitalization. Regardless of the kind of health care facility or of the type of health care sought, the client has preconceived ideas and feelings about each encounter with a health problem.

Whatever the experience, whether his own or the result of "second-hand" accounts, it influences the client's perception and expectations for the present situation. If the experience was threatening or unpleasant, the client may understandably fear the present situation. On the other hand, if the previous encounter was pleasant and rewarding, the client has expectations that may or may not be met in the present situation. In any event, the nurse needs to know how the client views his previous experiences so that his desires as well as his impressions can be incorporated into his plan of care. Such information may also tell the nurse something about the client's interpretation of a nurse's role and therefore help the nurse handle possible potential conflicts.

The client's expectations not only determine his behavior but influence his ability to accept or reject the plan of care. The client's response to his past experiences with health problems gives clues to his willingness to follow the present health regimen, his attitude toward health personnel, his methods of coping with stress, and his need for more information.

Asking about past experiences with illness or hospitalization lets the client know that the nurse is involved, that the nurse is interested in planning care that will include his needs and wishes, and that the nurse considers his feelings. Such a step helps establish open communication between client and nurse and will help develop trust—two vital components in the client-nurse relationship.

Level of knowledge and how the client interprets his health problems, diagnosis, and therapeutic regimen. The client's level of knowledge determines his understanding of his health problem, the prognosis, and the plan of care. How he interprets what he knows determines his acceptance of the problem, the prognosis and the plan of care, and influences the goals he establishes for himself. If the client understands the problem and accepts the prognosis and the plan of care, he will more than likely establish realistic objectives and goals. On the other hand, if the client does not understand his health problem or is confused about the plan of care, his goals become unrealistic and impossible to achieve. Mr. Weeks, a 60-year-old man, is admitted to the hospital with a diagnosis of cancer of the lung. He is scheduled for x-ray therapy once daily. When the nurse is taking the nursing history, Mr. Weeks states that he came to the hospital for a few days to have some tests done. The nurse calls the physician to tell him about Mr. Weeks's statement and to determine what Mr. Weeks had been told. The physician tells the nurse that x-ray therapy has been explained to Mr. Weeks and that he had agreed to the therapy plan. The nurse is now alert to a possible nursing problem. Further assessment will determine if Mr. Weeks is, in fact, denying the plan of therapy, is confused about the therapeutic regimen, or misunderstands the use of the term "x-ray."

Sometimes a misunderstanding concerning prognosis can delay therapy or seriously harm the client. For example, a young girl, after having reached puberty, had considerable bleeding with each menstrual period. After a diagnostic work-up it was determined she had a rare blood disease that required continual vigilance and periodic blood replacement. While living with her parents the girl faithfully followed the rigid therapeutic plan; but, believing maturity was correcting the problem and because she was bleeding less, she did not seek continued health care when she moved to another city. The first month away from home she bled rather severely with her menstrual period. The second month she bled so profusely that she was admitted to the hospital in deep shock and in critical condition. Because no one knew of her condition, it was some time before proper and complete therapy was determined and instigated.

Thorough and complete explanation is essential if the client is to accept and follow the therapeutic regimen. Often it is the nurse who must explain and help the client to understand, accept, and follow the plan of therapy. To do this the nurse must keep in close communication with the physician and other involved paramedical persons. Explanations need to be geared to the level of the client's understanding. Words, diagrams, and interpretations need to be within the client's frame of reference so that he will be able to understand and utilize the information.

Occupational and social roles. Illness, health care, and hospitalization in particular alter social and occupational roles. The usual patterns of daily living are often modified when the client is hospitalized, required to stay in bed, or limited in activity. Cardiac problems, diabetes, circulatory problems, and pregnancy are a few health conditions that alter a person's life style, which in turn may precipitate changes in the social and occupational roles. Awareness of the effect these roles have on the health situation or of how a health problem affects their role helps the individual cope more effectively during a crisis of the condition. Furthermore, the nurse needs to determine the method utilized by the client to cope with the needed changes. Sometimes the change is so drastic that the client is unable to cope with it. The client's ability to handle his health problem is often determined by his ability to adjust to its impact on his occupational role. A man who is able to leave work knowing that the job will be his when he returns is able to concentrate his energies on the task of acquiring health care. But the man who is preoccupied with the fear of losing his job if he remains away from it too long or by the fear that his health problem will alter his ability to handle the job, has little energy to tackle the chore of resolving the health problem.

Sometimes the occupational role of the client dictates the type of therapeutic plan. If the occupational role, for example, is one that requires the individual's attention and the treatment plan can be accomplished on an outpatient basis, then to hospitalize the client would create a new problem rather than alleviate the present health problem. More and more frequently day care or night care is available to those individuals seeking psychiatric care as options to complete hospitalization. X-ray therapy, diagnostic work-ups, and rehabilitative therapy are also available on a "drop-in" clinic-type basis.

Even if the individual is hospitalized, his plan of care needs to reflect his need for social interaction. Scheduling that indiscriminately denies the client's need for socialization hampers progress. Diagnostic tests and x-ray therapy should be scheduled so that the client has free time for family and friends.

At times the nursing problem centers around diminished family or visitor contact. A sense of loneliness coupled with the distress and uncertainty of illness often creates very stressful situations. Diminished social contact also deprives the nurse of additional resources for data collection about the client. Assisting the client to cope with loneliness and limited social contacts is therefore a vital part of nursing care. Developing the ability to utilize the client as the main source of data collection requires that the nurse be alert, sensitive, a good listener, and a capable interviewer.

A comprehensive nursing history that provides the nurse and other members of the health team with the client's occupational and social patterns contributes to a total assessment of the client's needs or problems.

Educational and intellectual capacity. Educational and intellectual capacity refers to the client's ability to comprehend and handle the events that affect his health. His ability to relate cause and effect, to evaluate and make decisions, and to understand his health status influences the client's degree of involvement in the plan of care. An assessment of the client's educational and intellectual capacity facilitates the establishment of a relevant and appropriate nursing approach. Teaching material that is beyond the comprehension of the client or his family only confuses and complicates the care plan. Teaching plans that are designed to meet the client's learning capacity go a long way toward increasing his awareness of the situation and his desire to be involved.

When interviewing the client and his family for the nursing history, the nurse uses the opportunity to assess their intellectual capacity. Are they aware of what is happening? Are their questions pertinent to the situation? Does their language use seem consistent with their educational preparation? Can they solve problems? Do they assume responsibility for and consider the plan of care as their concern? Are they able to assimilate and integrate the physician's explanations? Have they a realistic appraisal of the health picture? Have they established objectives or goals for the future? Do they understand the plan of care?

An evaluation of the client's intellectual ability and his educational preparation determines how much and in what way the client can be informed about his health problem and plan of care. Knowledge of the intellectual capacity of the client and of his educational preparation allows the nurse to plan care, to make explanations, and to expect involvement, which are neither beyond his ability nor demeaning to him.

Recreational, religious, and health practices. Recreational customs, religious practices, and preferred health care play a major part in nursing care planning. Knowledge of the individual's religious practices allows the nurse to order appropriate diets, to make arrangements for specific rituals, and to be sensitive to the customs that are so much a part of the client's life. Perhaps the client in the hospital is a Catholic and wishes to receive daily communion. In such case the priest should be notified and the night staff should be alerted so the client can be prepared in the early morning for the priest's visit. If the client is Jewish and wishes to observe dietary restrictions, the dietician must be informed. If the client is a Jehovah's Witness, appropriate communication with the staff, physician, and all concerned is necessary to acknowledge and respect the client's desire to avoid blood transfusions.

Recreational practices often are the client's means of promoting better health. The daily golf game, the weekly bowling game, or a daily tennis match are often the client's way of obtaining exercise and mental or emotional renewal. Illness, restricted activity, or potential health problems may interfere or suddenly halt such practices. These activities are important items for the nurse to know so that appropriate scheduling for outpatient therapy or diversive activities for inpatient care can be incorporated into the plan of care.

A rule of thumb that helps the nurse in assessing health problems to determine the appropriate plan of care is to remember always to "maximize the client's strengths and to minimize his weaknesses." At all times the nurse needs to assess the client for areas in which the plan of care can best make use of the client's already established patterns of health care. If the client exercises each morning before breakfast by running for thirty minutes, then whenever possible this activity should be included in his daily schedule. If such a strenuous activity is not possible, a substitute activity can be found. If the client is accustomed to eating light suppers but enjoys a hearty lunch, this routine should be incorporated into his plan of care whenever possible.

Language usage. Language is the universal means of communicating. Yet the use of language often creates communication problems. Misunderstood terms, medical jargon, and private words are only a few of the reasons for confusion. To the sophisticated hospitalized client, such terms as "void," "catheterize," "hypo," and "sleeper" make sense. But to the neophyte they are mystifying. Medical jargon, such as N.P.O., $\overline{ac}$, $\overline{pc}$, intake and output, diastolic and systolic pressure, percussion, auscultation, and so on, are words or symbols that have no meaning for the average person and that tend to separate the client from the events that are occurring to him or within him. On the other hand, private terms that have particular significance for the client have little meaning to others. Colloquial words for the parts of the body or for the elimination processes are common. Pet names for loved ones, slang terms, and cultural jargon are some of the areas that need clarification.

Data about the client's vocabulary, his ability to send and receive messages, are important to the plan of care. Such problems as stuttering, deafness, foreign language usage, language deficiencies because of different cultural experiences, all limit the expression and the comprehension of communication. During the history taking the nurse notes whether the client's or the family's responses convey any problems in understanding or expression and whether they are the result of a language barrier.

Economic status and employment patterns. The economic status of the client tells the nurse something about his style of life as well as the degree of his economic security. Individuals who have economic problems are often preoccupied with worry about the cost of the health care and whether the family can manage under the added strain of health expense. History has demonstrated that in times of depression, health care receives low priority. In times of economic stress the client often limits his hospital stay, returning to work earlier than is advisable. Nursing care for these individuals should include teaching the client about follow-up care as well as care that is designed especially for his short stay.

An individual's life style often is a reflection of his economic status. If the individual is accustomed to gourmet meals, wine, and candlelight, then such practices need to be known so that measures may be taken to accommodate such customs as soon as possible, as determined by the situation. Perhaps the meals or the atmosphere will not be exactly as desired, but at least the client is aware that the plan of care is attempting to meet his needs.

At the other end of the spectrum is the individual who never really is sure about his next meal or his housing arrangements. These persons are frequently hoarders of food. They eat all they can and also store some of their food for a time in the future. Such practices are sources of problems and need direct identification and clarification so that other alternatives can be devised that (1) offer the client greater security, (2) offer long-range solutions, and (3) provide necessary nourishment. For instance, is the client aware that frequent or between-meal snacks are available or that social welfare programs or job opportunity programs exist? Once again the nurse's awareness of such behavior allows for inclusion of meals that meet the individual's needs in the care plan and referral to the proper sources for follow-up care.

Level of behavioral growth and development. Knowledge of normal behavioral growth and development is an essential tool when assessing needs. Baseline behavioral criteria provide the nurse with a measuring device for determining nursing problems. Being able to distinguish normal dependency needs from abnormal needs for any particular age level helps the nurse identify a problem. For instance, knowing that adolescence is a stage of identity crisis in which the individual is seeking, testing, and demanding independence enables the nurse to handle the adolescent client who is hostile, demanding, and often contradictory in his behavior. School, public health, and psychiatric nurses are often involved in interactions with adolescents and their parents. An assessment based on observations and interviews with family and client helps the nurse establish the adolescent's behavior on the dependent-independent continuum and determine what steps to take.

A determination of the behavioral development of a child gives the nurse critical information for planning hospital care. Knowing that separation anxiety is often the response of a 2-year-old child helps the nurse plan for the child's adjustment to the hospital. Information that tells the nurse how the child was prepared and what the child was told guides the nurse in planning care that helps alleviate the child's anxiety.

Awareness of the 2-year-old's behavioral development also alerts the nurse to the child's need to assert his autonomy. The nurse who plans care for the 2-year-old will need to consider how to handle his negativistic behavior. Information from the mother about the child's toilet training, language development, appetite demands, and disciplinary needs enables the nurse to plan nursing care specifically for the 2-year-old child.

At the other extreme are the effects of aging on the individual's response to illness. Impaired vision, deafness, and limited mobility often interfere with or compound the elderly person's adjustment to hospitalization. One response often seen with elderly persons is regression, that is, a return to earlier modes of behavior to handle stress They may cry, have temper tantrums, pout, wet the bed, or adopt other childlike behavior to handle the stress of illness. Some of this response is physiologically oriented but a great deal is a regressive adaptation. An understanding of the elderly individual's regressive behavior allows the nursing staff to plan ways to help the individual cope more appropriately with the stress of his health problem.

How the individual perceives himself and how he accepts his aging process greatly influence his adaptation to and involvement in his plan of care. Those persons who see themselves as useful and productive individuals, regardless of age, tend to become involved in their plan of care and actively seek maximum health. Those who see themselves as useless and deteriorating individuals develop many and varied nursing problems.

No matter what the chronological age, the individual's response to his health problem is affected by his level of behavioral development. Therefore to develop individualized nursing care specific information about the person's behavioral development is required.

Present and past coping behaviors utilized for handling stress. Data on the client's past coping patterns is crucial information, when attempting to plan therapeutic intervention. Information is sought to determine what strengths the individual has, what coping skills he may have used successfully in the past, and what resources he utilized to help him cope with situations.

As the nurse gathers data about the client's coping behaviors, certain questions come to mind. What were the first symptoms to be noticed and what did the client do about them? Did he try to handle things by himself? Did he ignore the symptoms? When did he seek professional help? Did he follow the professional advice? If not, why not? How did the family react to his health problem? What are his goals for the treatment plan? These questions and others give the nurse a general picture of the client's pattern of behavior when faced with a health crisis. They also determine the extent of family disruption and how it was handled.

The client's ability to cope with the present health problem is determined by three factors:

1. Past success with his present coping patterns
2. The extent of stress evoked by the present situation
3. His ability to devise and implement new coping behaviors when necessary

The nurse needs to identify all three factors when planning care, since an assessment of the individual's coping behaviors frequently determines areas of deficiency and a need for teaching. Some coping behaviors need support, that is, they need to be maintained and strengthened. Others need to be corrected, since they have become malfunctioning or maladaptive. Other coping behaviors need to be created, since they are nonexistent. The type of nursing intervention depends on an accurate appraisal of the client's coping potential.

Usual cultural patterns of daily living. Patterns of daily living, such as food preferences and eating habits, hygienic and sleep patterns, and elimination routines play a major role in everyday lives. Disruption by illness, health care, and hospitalization often creates a need to change and to adapt to other established institutional routines. Whether the health care is in a hospital, a clinic, or a home, it often necessitates a change in the preferred acts of daily living.

Food and eating habits are highly individualized. They are the result of cultural, ethnic, and social customs and are influenced by occupation, social status, and geographic area. Food intake is for more than sustenance, it is also an important means of social interaction and pleasurable self-gratification. Eating removes the pain of hunger and satisfies the sensual needs of taste, smell, and sight. Therefore, to alter a person's diet is to tamper with a major part of his personal and social gratification. Dietary matters form an important area for inclusion in the nursing history.

The act of tasting, smelling, and viewing food is the basis for food likes and dislikes. Too often clients on diets must eat foods that are rich in vitamins and minerals but that for one reason or another are not liked. Prompt attention by the nurse to discover the client's likes and dislikes not only saves much unpleasantness but communicates concern and improves nutrition. An awareness of the client's likes and dislikes can also indicate areas of nutritional deficiency and therefore has teaching implications for the nurse.

Eating habits include the time for eating, the usual foods taken at each meal, and the type of social interaction that accompanies the meal. Work schedules often determine the time and the content of meals. Take, for example, Mr. Klein, who has worked as a security guard from twelve noon to twelve midnight for the past 10 years. He usually has a hearty breakfast at ten in the morning and a hot dinner at a local restaurant at five in the evening, at which time he enjoys the company of several truck drivers who patronize the establishment. When he arrives home at midnight he has a snack and a bottle of beer before retiring. Recently Mr. Klein was diagnosed hypertensive and overweight and was placed on a 1000-calorie diet and instructed to exercise three times a day. To minimize the disruption of his already well-established eating routine, the nurse needs to help Mr. Klein alter the quality and quantity of his present diet to fit the prescribed diet and yet maintain his schedule. To expect Mr. Klein to change the time, the content, and the place at which he eats is to expect unrealistic change. He can learn to alter the caloric intake of his diet, to eat less, and yet continue to enjoy the company of his buddies at the restaurant.

If Mr. Klein becomes hospitalized, some major changes in meal timing will be necessary. The concerned nurse could help him select low-calorie foods that he likes and could provide social interaction. The nurse either facilitates social interaction between Mr. Klein and his roommates or, if he is in a private room, suggests he invite his family and friends to dine with him. More and more frequently hospitals are providing dining rooms where the ambulatory patients can eat, converse, and socialize.

It would be important to alert the hospital staff to Mr. Klein's unusual working hours so that they would not be confused by his seemingly bizarre sleeping pattern and desire to eat at different times from the hospital routine.

Of course, if the individual wishes to eat alone his wishes should be respected. Privacy can be established if the nurse is aware of the need. Private rooms, screens, or curtains are a few of the ways to provide quiet and privacy during mealtime.

An area of most frequent concern to hospitalized clients is the type of atmosphere provided at mealtime. Odors, unpleasant sights, and disagreeable procedures all too frequently disturb mealtime. The sensitive and aware nurse can provide a quiet and attractive mealtime environment. Blood-stained dressings, half-full drainage bottles, urinals, and bedpans, should be placed out of sight. Odors from dressings, urine collectors, drainage bottles, and colostomy receptacles can be reduced with deoderizers, adequate ventilation, and judicious removal or frequent emptying. Procedures can be scheduled to avoid mealtimes. Certainly the practice of providing a clean and pleasant environment is essential when the client's appetite is poor.

Other areas that need consideration when planning nursing care are hygienic practices and sleep patterns. Bathing and grooming habits are an integral part of the acts of daily living and are therefore important areas to be evaluated by the nurse. Determining the preference of type and time for such practices is essential if individualized care is the goal. Traditionally, the institution determines the bathing routine; but with a little flexibility and ingenuity the situation can be changed. Personal preference sheets (check lists) are easily developed and can be part of the admission routine. Whether the client bathes once a day, twice a week, or weekly depends on his need and desire and not on staffing availability or agency policy. The client and his family can be included in hygienic care decisions and in implementation. Changes in bathing routines, like any other changes, occur when there is a need. When nurses identify needs, changes are possible. Individualized care demands that traditional routines be critically reassessed and that nursing care become a function for meeting client needs rather than rituals of practice.

The discomfort of illness and therapy coupled with worry over the health problem and its impact tend to make sleep difficult. Yet adequate sleep and rest are important elements of the healing process. Many factors contribute to the ability to sleep. Such things as the sleep environment and the usual methods employed to induce sleep influence the ability or inability to get to sleep and stay asleep. Environmental considerations include temperature, light, noise, privacy, and type of bed, blankets, and pillows. If the individual is accustomed to sleeping in a room with the door closed, with a small night light turned on, and with the windows open 3 inches from the top, this information needs to be included in the nursing care plan. Each person has his own idiosyncracies about the sleeping room. The number of blankets, number and position of pillows, and the type of mattress all contribute to comfort and need to be known and implemented to deter sleeping problems. Noise and light (unless otherwise indicated) should be kept to a minimum. A well-ventilated but not drafty room eliminates the stuffy and congested feeling so often found in the sickroom.

Of prime consideration is the means by which each individual either promotes sleep or handles sleeplessness. Too often nurses administer sleeping medication to the hospital client who is having difficulty sleeping without first trying other means. Warm baths, warm beverages, soft music, repositioning, or back rubs frequently induce sleep. An inquiry into the client's preference helps establish relevant and appropriate approaches.

No discussion of the patterns of daily living is complete without mention of elimination routines. Information about the client's usual bowel behavior provides the nurse with baseline knowledge. This knowledge helps the nurse determine progress, identify learning needs, and discover problems. For instance, knowledge of Mrs. Lawler's daily use of laxatives to promote bowel evacuation enables the nurse to plan nursing care that incorporates this practice. Mrs. Lawler's expectation of a daily bowel movement is reflective of a culture that is very bowel conscious. Even so, for some people a bowel movement once every two or three days is sufficient. In either case the nurse needs to know the client's attitude and routine so that fears can be alleviated, problems can be avoided, and individualized attention can be guaranteed.

Problems with urinary elimination are also important data for the nursing history. If Mrs. Lawler tells the nurse that she has always had frequent voiding and often urinates several times in the night, such information needs to be communicated to all others involved in her care, so that these behaviors are not mistaken for indication of an acute urinary problem, when in fact they are part of Mrs. Lawler's normal urinary behavior.

Many other areas of daily living might be discussed here but because the acts of eating, sleeping, and eliminating are universal they have been covered. The nurse should also elicit information about the client's hobbies and activities or other interests that might influence or affect nursing care.

Relationships with significant others. Every individual has some one or more persons in whom he confides, from whom he seeks advice, or to whom he looks for guidance. These confidants or counselors play an important role in helping the client maintain or promote optimal health and in alleviating health problems. When decisions need to be made, information verified, bad news delivered, or support provided, this significant person is called upon. The nurse needs to know of this person or persons and sometimes needs to involve them in decisions concerning the client if health teaching, changes in attitudes and practices, consent, or involvement in therapy are to be accomplished.

Obviously the amount and the type of information included in the nursing history is determined by the client, his problem, the type of care sought, and the philosophy of the agency. Not all nursing histories include all the areas discussed. Selection of area of inquiry is determined by the relevance of that area to the health situation. To determine relevancy the nurse might list and check off each area mentioned until the pertinent and usable areas are identified.

Nursing history and the community

To this point the nursing history has been related to the individual or the family. The nursing history of a community is similar but different, too. Community health problems are in effect people problems, so in this context the nurse is again assessing the needs of the individual. But community health nursing is not only responsible for developing and maintaining individual health; it is also concerned with the social well-being of all the members of the community. Nurses therefore assess community health needs by developing a nursing history of the community. They assess the community by collecting data about the community's problems. Data on the unemployed, the number of pathogenic diseases, the available parks and recreational facilities, the adequacy of sewage and garbage collection, and the availability of schools, as well as many other factors, are collected, compiled, and indexed. It is from these indices that interpretations are made and used as a basis for action.

Nurses also assess individual needs as a means of identifying community problems. An example may help clarify this point. A teenage boy of 18 seeks medical advice from the school nurse about clinical symptoms that he believes indicate venereal disease. The nurse refers the boy to a physician who confirms the boy's suspicions and begins treatment. In addition to treating the boy, the physician reports the case to the public health department, since epidemiological measures must be carried out if the venereal disease is to be controlled effectively. Few physicians have the staff or the time to carry out an epidemiological survey. Also, it is considered a community-centered rather than a person-centered activity, and is therefore best performed by a public health agency—the agency whose primary concern is the whole community.

The epidemiological investigation begins with the collection of data about the identified client and his contacts. The public health nurse not only assesses the boy's needs by developing a nursing history in order to assist the physician in formulating a plan of care, but also repeats this process with each contact to determine what health needs each one has.

The ultimate result of this example might be the discovery that one of the problems is a lack of community awareness about venereal disease. One nursing action might be to propose to the school districts, where the highest incidence of venereal disease is present, that they instigate an educational program to inform the public of the incidence, transmission, clinical symptoms, and ultimate consequences of venereal disease. The public health nurse might act as consultant to the school nurse to develop the program.

Community health problems are the responsibility of nurses wherever they choose to work, whether hospital, clinic, physician's office, industry, or public health agency. All nurses are involved in the health care of the community. But an assessment of the community's health needs is the responsibility of the public health agency. Reporting of communicable health problems by the physician and the nurse to the public health agency alerts the agency to potential community health problems. Demographic surveys, which statistically study those factors affecting health and mortality, are then utilized by the public health agency to pinpoint the area and individuals involved. The results of these studies often lead to the formulation of health programs that control disease, promote health, and prevent illness. Public health nurses are involved, by the nature of their skill in observation and interviewing, in demographic surveys. Their prime goal is to determine the nursing needs of the individual within the context of his family and the community.

Past experiences with health problems, the level of knowledge, and intellectual capacity of those involved would be assessed to determine learning needs. The economic, social, and ethnic background of all concerned would be assessed to determine their cultural response to the situation. How each affected person copes with the health problem and how collectively they respond to health care need to be evaluated. And above all, knowing who are the accepted, respected, and influential leaders of the community is essential if the health program is to be accepted and implemented.

METHODS OF GATHERING DATA

Observations, interviews, diagnostic findings, and records supply the needed information for an assessment. Records and interviews with the client and his family or friends provide the nursing history. Observations and a clinical evaluation of the client's present behavior provide baseline data for a complete assessment and for measuring changes. Observations of the client include an inspection of the client's general appearance, his interpersonal interactions, his motor activity and his body language, his home, his friends and family, and his community. Observation of the family tells the nurse something about the type of family structure, the strengths of the family, the coping patterns of the family unit, and the relationship control of the family. Observations of the community situation tell the nurse where the health problem exists, who is affected by the health problem, and what the effect or consequence of the health problem may be.

Observation and clinical evaluation

Observation is a descriptive, not an interpretive or evaluative, act. It is made by using the five senses: sight, smell, touch, taste, and hearing. Observation is influenced by the observer's past experiences and ability to be thorough, his ability to pick up subtle clues, and his ability to remain objective.

A clinical evaluation is the process of interpreting what has been observed. The observable data are compared to a norm and are found to be either within or outside normal limits. The clinical evaluation also notes the presence or absence of certain conditions.

General appearance. The general appearance of the client, the family, or the community tells the nurse much about the general health of each. During the first encounter with the client the nurse begins the observational inspection. By viewing the individual the nurse can determine any grossly apparent abnormalities. On further examination, a notation should be made about the color, texture, and appearance of the skin; the condition of the teeth, oral mucosa, muscle tone, and the joint range of motion; the color of the sclera, nail beds, lips, and extremities; the rate, rhythm, and character of respirations and pulse; temperature of the skin and the odor of the client's breath, skin, and clothes.

Part of the nurse's observations should include the client's tone of voice, use of eye contact, and manner of dress. Evidence of edema, lesions, skin eruptions, bleeding, pain, and trauma should be recorded.

During the clinical evaluation, the nurse takes the blood pressure, temperature, height, weight, and neurological signs. These measurements together with the observed phenomena provide a composite picture of the client, which can be compared to clinical or theoretical norms to determine deviations. They also provide a reference point for future evaluation. The end result of such a process is a descriptive evaluation of the client's general health status. Information from further diagnostic tests, interviews, and past health records is necessary to complete the assessment.

When gathering data about the general appearance of a family, the nurse observes the composition and the health of the family. Who are its members? How many children are there? What are the members' approximate ages? What sex are they? What is each member's general health appearance? If the nurse can visit the family's home, a description of the neighborhood and the house helps the nurse gain information about their socioeconomic level and their values. A neat, well-kept house and yard in a low-income neighborhood may indicate the family is poor but socially conscientious. Supportive evidence from interviews is necessary before an evaluation and interpretation of the observed data is possible.

Much information can be obtained by observing the general appearance of a community. Again, the nurse may be placed in a position in which the appearance of a community is critical to the indentification of a health problem. Astute and precise reporting of what is seen, touched, and smelled is essential to accurate assessment. The nurse should describe the location, size, and state of housing available. Some pertinent questions are: Who lives there? How many live in each dwelling? Are there ample toilet and refuse facilities? Is there running water? A description of the recreational and transportation facilities and the proximity of business gives added data for making a community assessment.

Interpersonal interaction. Observing the client's interpersonal behavior tells the nurse about his patterns of socialization, his anxiety level, his acceptance or rejection of his health problem, and his general ability to cope with the present situation. An evaluation of this observable data clues the nurse to appropriate or inappropriate coping behaviors and therefore to the areas that need reinforcement and the areas that need to be changed. The nurse may also discover who is significant in the client's life and something about his decision-making skills, while observing his interpersonal behavior.

Careful listening coupled with a knowledge of ethnicity allows the nurse to determine different cultural responses and patterns of behavior that are significant to particular social and ethnic groups. An awareness of such responses or patterns of behavior is important when planning individualized nursing care.

When observing the interpersonal interaction of a family, it helps to view the unit in totality. Is the family a matriarchal or patriarchal unit? Perhaps the most significant clues to the relationship control of the family may be found in discovering the member who identifies the problem, who is looked upon by the others for answers or support, and who seems to make the decisions. The nurse needs to look critically at the roles each member plays. Are the parents assuming the role of adult? Of parent? Or do they look to the child for guidance and direction? Assumed roles by any member tells a lot about the relationship of the family and a great deal about how they will react to outside help. Observations of the family's configuration and of its role assignments reveal as much about the family as a temperature chart discloses about the individual. Many families under stress react to form a close unit while others split and fragment. An observation of the family members in action, that is, how they relate to one another, often tells the nurse something about their ability to cope with the health problem and with one another.

Motor activity. The client's motor activity should be observed. His agility, his range of motion, his ability to manage himself are all indications of his place on the dependence-independence continuum. Limitations in motor functioning need to be evaluated to determine in what areas the client needs assistance.

> Mr. Stanton, a 67-year-old man, suffered from chronic osteoarthritis and was unable to lift either of his hands to his face to feed himself. His clever son designed and constructed a device that, when strapped to his right arm, enabled him to feed himself. When taking the nursing history on his admission to the hospital, the nurse noticed his inability to lift and bend his arms. This astute observation prompted the nurse to ask pertinent questions and thus to learn about his unique eating apparatus.

Because the nurse inquired about what she saw, care was planned to meet the client's needs.

Motor limitations exist for most aged individuals. The inability of the aged to manage alone in the bathtub or shower, to navigate in and out of bed, and to move about freely and without pain are just a few of the motor limitations that need to be considered when planning care.

Small children have motor and safety needs that demand consideration when planning nursing care. Can the child manage safely in a crib when he is ill? Does he need a protective fence across the door of his room? Can he handle the available toys safely when confined to a crib or his room when sick? Is the child at the level of motor development that is within normal limits for his age? These and many other questions enter the nurse's mind when observing the child at play and evaluating the child's level of activity.

Body language.. Along with an awareness of the client's motor activity, observation of his body language lets the nurse know how he uses his body to communicate his needs. By definition[2] body language means the behavioral patterns the client uses to communicate nonverbal messages. Many messages that individuals convey are sent by gestures, body position, and a mixture of body movements. Stance, distance relationship, facial expressions, and posture tell much about how the client feels. With advancing age it becomes more difficult to hide feelings or to pretend. Faces droop, bodies sag, and frowns do not fade away.

Body language is particularly significant when the client becomes mute. For although a person may stop talking, he does not stop communicating. In fearful situations hands shake and legs tremble. In painful situations faces become tense and the body becomes rigid. And when a person is happy, his whole body lets the world know. The real value of body language, however, remains in its blending with the spoken word to convey thoughts, ideas, and feelings.

The preceding section has introduced many areas that need to be observed when making an assessment for the plan of care for a client. But in no way is it a complete list. Each unique situation prescribes observational possibilities. It is up to the nurse, skilled in observational techniques, to notice those items, expressions, and happenings that are pertinent and significant.

Interviewing

To assess the needs of the client the nurse uses not only observation skills but also develops the ability to communicate in such a way that the client understands what is said, the nurse understands what the client is saying, and the health team comprehends what both are saying. Communication involves a sender, a message, and a receiver. The cycle may be considered complete when the message is understood by the receiver in the approximate manner in which the sender intended.[3] The message may be considered incomplete when the receiver derives a meaning other than that intended by the sender. In the nursing situation the client and nurse are both viewed alternately as sender and receiver. The client-sender relays a message to the nurse-receiver who then sends a response to the client or carries the message to other

---

[2] Fast, Julius: Body language, Philadelphia, 1970, J. B. Lippincott Co., p. 9.

[3] Ruesch, Jurgen: Therapeutic communication, New York, 1961, W. W. Norton & Company, Inc., pp. 452-455.

members of the health team. In this complex cycle many factors either facilitate or detract from the communication. Such factors as (1) timing, (2) fatigue, (3) distractions, (4) disruptions, and (5) motivation influence the nurse-client interaction.

The time at which the interview is planned as well as the length of time spent in the interview is important. Ideally an interview to gather data for the nursing history occurs soon after the client seeks health care. Obviously there are exceptions to this statement. For example, individuals in crisis situations need immediate health care and are therefore not available for an interview. Unconscious persons, persons with language barriers, or sedated and disoriented persons cannot participate in an interview. In these instances the nurse gathers data from others until the client is able to participate. However, when the client cannot participate in the interview, data from relatives, records, and observation suffice.

The length of time needed to acquire a nursing history during an interview depends on many factors. The content, the interpersonal environment, the client's willingness to participate, the verbosity of the client, the skill of the nurse, and the complexity of the health problem are just a few of the factors. The experienced and skilled interviewer can conduct an interview and collect the needed data in 15 to 20 minutes. The secret to success lies in the nurse's ability to guide the client through the process, keeping communication open and yet not letting the client ramble.

During the interview emotional areas may arise and tempt the nurse to begin therapy. This may or may not be the time to handle the problem. It will depend on the amount of time available to the nurse, the degree of concern the client expresses, the relationship the concern has to the client's health problem, and the amount of data collected. Perhaps the nurse has enough data to begin a plan of care and can therefore intervene appropriately. On the other hand, if the nurse has insufficient data with which to make a valid and safe decision, stopping the client and asking a few pertinent and vital questions enables the nurse to gather needed data to intervene.

The fatigue level of the client needs to be considered also. Sometimes even 15 minutes is too long for critically ill or highly emotional persons to spend in an interview. The nurse needs to critically observe the client and terminate the interview if fatigue is apparent. A point to remember is that not all the nursing history needs to come from the client, nor is all of the information needed initially. Perhaps more than one interview will be necessary before a complete nursing history is obtained.

Freedom from distraction is essential to the success of the interview. Pain, noise, and preoccupation with worry or fear create barriers to the nurse-client interaction. The distraction of pain means that the client directs most of his energy toward his discomfort and has little available energy for discussion. The nurse who sees that the client is free of pain and is comfortable finds that he is not only willing to participate but is also able to get more fully involved in the interchange.

Disruptions caused by noise or extreme activity break the continuity of the interaction and demand that the interviewer compete for the client's attention. Preoccupation with worry or fear creates the same sort of situation. Skilled nurse interaction encourages the client to express his worries and fears in an attempt to reduce the distraction and to help the client explore his concerns. And the interviewer who plans for privacy reduces the chance of noise distraction.

Motivation influences the quantity and the quality of the nurse-client communication. Since motivation is a factor of need, the client will be motivated to communicate when he perceives a need. Most persons are willing to give information and to become involved in their plan of care. Refusal or reluctance during an interview may occur. If it does the nurse tries to determine the cause of the client's nonresponse. Nonverbal communication is as important as verbal communication and often leads to the discovery of deep feelings. If the client seems reluctant or is embarrassed, the nurse attempts to convey a patient and accepting manner. The nurse might postpone the interview or collect the needed information from other sources or might respond to the client's nonverbal behavior in a supportive manner.

Barriers to effective communication. Problems in communication may arise from:

1. Illness of the client
2. Differences in age and experience of nurse and client
3. The psychological development of the client and of the nurse
4. Differences in the client's and nurse's cultural, social, and ethnic backgrounds
5. Differences between nurse's and client's expectations

Resolution of these problems can be approached through the use of an open and supportive interchange of ideas, feelings, and expectations. The establishment of a trust relationship is essential if a therapeutic relationship between the client and the nurse is to be formed. Trust in the client will help the nurse to accept him as a unique and valuable individual. In the nurse-client relationship, trust is a mutual expectation of the essential reliability of each member. Skill in the ability to recognize one's own inner feelings allows the nurse to tap the interpersonal atmosphere by the personal awareness of the impact of the interchange. Many communicative problems can be avoided if the nurse listens, observes, and attempts to understand nonverbal messages by clarifying and validating assumptions. Misunderstandings in communication can be resolved when the nurse validates feelings and clarifies incongruent messages.

Purposes of the interview. How an interview is defined and conducted is directly related to the goals of each nursing episode. However, there are a

common core of purposes for all interviews. These purposes are:
1. To help establish interpersonal relationships
2. To provide clients with an opportunity to ventilate and explore their feelings
3. To gather information about the client to determine a plan of care

There are many types of interviews; far too many to discuss all of them here. How the interview proceeds depends largely on the nurse's purpose, the client's problem, and the philosophy of the agency. Regardless of any of these factors, nurses must remember to keep the lines of communication open.

There are many ways of keeping communication open. The use of open-ended questions, incomplete sentences, paraphrasing, reflection, and nonverbal gesturing serve the purpose. The temptation to cut off the client's verbalization with reassurance or by focusing on specific information the nurse wants to obtain must be resisted or delayed. Words or voice tones that imply "everything will be all right" can close off communication. Giving the client verbal and nonverbal reinforcement to continue keeps the communication open.

A major function of the nurse in the role of interviewer is to promote client participation. Minimal verbal activity combined with nonverbal activity is probably the best approach to encouragement of client expression. But this is not simple. Silence makes most people uncomfortable and can therefore give rise to an increase in the nurse's verbal behavior. As the nurse's verbal activity increases, the client's activity is reduced. But if the nurse remains quiet, conveys by body movement and position her concern, interest and attention, then the client will respond. Nodding the head, saying "Go on," and leaning forward as if anticipating, and saying "Tell me about . . . " are examples of behaviors the nurse might employ as means of encouraging the client to respond. A productive interview is one in which the client's production is high and the nurse's activity is low.

Focusing directs the interview. Focusing is indicating topics to be discussed based on the client's stated concerns. It produces information relevant to the stated problem areas. Responding to leads and clues provided by the client allows the nurse to direct the interview. The nurse needs to be aware of the client's many verbal and nonverbal clues—his body tension, sudden stops, change in voice tone, recurrent themes—to be able to focus. Too little focusing creates a "chit-chat" session, while too much direction can create a highly structured question-and-answer time in which the nurse gets information but the client has little chance to vent feelings or to develop any relationship with the nurse. Focus produces direction, but does not stifle exploration. When the nurse is alert to the client's concerns, knows how to follow a "train of thought," knows when a digression is "off course," the client can be directed toward sorting and problem solving. This type of sorting and decision making is vital if the interview is to be productive for both client and nurse.

Library resources

Gathering data for safe and appropriate problem identification and nursing intervention demands that the nurse and the nursing team utilize all possible resources. One very valuable resource is the library. No one can know enough to provide solutions to the many nursing problems encountered in hospitals, clinics, physician's offices, industries, or homes. Library research can provide current behavioral theories, new therapies, information about new drugs and diagnostic measures to increase the nurse's expertise in problem identification and nursing intervention.

When the nurse is baffled by a breakdown in communication, a trip to the library to read up on communication theory helps. New drugs, medical advances, and technological innovations generate the need for continued study. Keeping abreast of the knowledge explosion is a full-time job, but one that allows the nurse to offer the best nursing care possible to the client.

Since nursing is concerned with people and their health problems, an understanding of human behavior and man's reactions to his environment is essential. Nurses cannot function effectively without constantly being aware of and responding to changing social trends, such as the complex and unique responses of ethnic groups to health needs and care, and the impact of political and other pressure groups on health programs. The nurse who reads all types of literature (newspapers, professional journals, abstracts, popular periodicals, and textbooks) has information pertinent to the ever-changing social milieu and can therefore plan nursing care that provides for the complexities of the health problems of the modern client. Thus, as the nurse broadens her understanding of all phases of human behavoir, the nursing care becomes increasingly holistic.

Health records

To complete the data-gathering process, the nurse refers to the medical and social records. Valuable information is available to the nurse in these records. The medical record provides diagnostic results, progress notes, physical examination findings, consultation reports, and the medical history.

The social history provides information about the client's occupation, his economic standing, and something about his home life. Together, these two sources (1) supply the nurse with pertinent data for needed teaching, (2) alert the nurse to possible complications, and (3) verify the nurse's own observations.

In addition, information from the client's health records increases the nurse's awareness of the client's past response to health problems and gives the nurse a running account of what is happening currently, what progress, if any, the client is making, and what to expect.

COMPLETING THE ASSESSMENT

After the nurse has collected the needed data, the information is classified, analyzed, and summarized to complete the assessment. In other words, data concerned with any one particular area are grouped together and, by the process of inductive or deductive analysis, generalizations or hypotheses are formed, inferences are made, and speculations are proposed. These generalizations are then compared with clinical or theoretical norms to determine nursing problems.

The following section will demonstrate how the data collected are classified and analyzed to complete the assessment. Then, utilizing the stress-response model presented in Chapter Two, it will be shown how the assessment aids in identifying a nursing problem.

Classifying the data

Once the nurse has collected the available data, all information that pertains to any given area is placed together. Data from the client's social and occupational life are separated from data gained from laboratory tests. Data about the client's expectations and goals are placed together, whereas information concerning his level of understanding and intellectual capacity is placed in another category. This categorizing organizes data into logical areas for consideration. Without category grouping, the nurse would be faced with a hodgepodge of information that gives little or no meaning to identifying nursing problems, since each area is regarded as a potential problem area. For instance, all data concerning the client's or family's expectations, when analyzed, may indicate unrealistic expectations. Data from laboratory tests might determine imbalances or diagnose disease processes. It should be remembered that categorized data not only help identify health problems but aid in ruling out problems. For example, categorized data might appear as follows:

Personal characteristics	Social data	Medical data	Goals and expectations

Analysis of data

Following a classification of the data comes an analysis to complete the assessment. The data are examined in the light of their impact on the overall health of the individual, family, or community. It should also be determined via the assessment whether the problem has nursing implications. If no nursing implications exist, the nurse refers the client to the proper source.

An analysis of the classified data enables the nurse to determine the nature, significance, and relationship of one category to another to arrive at a conclusion. Utilizing deductive and inductive reasoning, generalizations are formed, which explain or predict relationships and from which problems are extracted. When the inductive process is used, generalizations are developed from a set of observations or facts. For instance, if the nurse observes the client (who is diagnosed as severely depressed because of the loss of employment) to be noncommunicative, anorexic, insomnic, and immobile, the generalization is that severely depressed individuals experience difficulty in maintaining the acts of daily living. The nurse's knowledge of the psychodynamics of depression verifies this generalization. From this generalization, nursing problems can be extracted. A comparison of this generalization with the knowledge that man needs food, sleep, social interaction, and activity to maintain health allows the nurse to identify health problems.

Inductive process

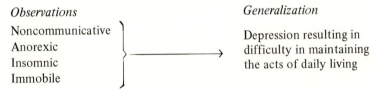

Observations

Noncommunicative
Anorexic
Insomnic
Immobile

Generalization

Depression resulting in difficulty in maintaining the acts of daily living

There are times when the assessment is developed from a deductive process. Suppose the nurse reads in the client's chart that he is immobile. Using the generalization that "immobility creates stasis in the circulatory and alimentary systems," the nurse hypothesizes that "immobile individuals develop constipation, lung congestion, and poor venous return." The cognitive process used in this example begins with a generalization and arrives at a conclusion, which is in itself a generalization. From this second generalization the hypothesized problems of lung congestion, poor venous return, and constipation need to be verified. Further data collection and comparison will either validate or rule out the problems.

Deductive process

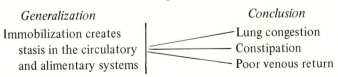

Generalization

Immobilization creates stasis in the circulatory and alimentary systems

Conclusion

Lung congestion
Constipation
Poor venous return

Assessment not only enables the nurse to identify nursing problems, it also supplies information for individualized nursing care. This kind of information is important in planning nursing care, but it does not point out nursing problems. For example, the nursing history indicates the client's food preferences. Knowing food preferences is important when planning nursing care but does not indicate a problem, unless the preferred food is contraindicated by the disease process or by the therapeutic regimen. Information regarding the client's patterns of daily living is the kind of data that helps the nurse adapt the nursing care to the individual desires of the client, but is not contributory to problem identification.

PROBLEM IDENTIFICATION

As stated in Chapter One, health problems exist when there is an unmet need and there is no unimpeded action possible to meet the need. Health problems arise when the client, family, or community:
1. Cannot meet a need
2. Needs help to meet a need
3. Is not aware of an unmet need
4. Has a conflict of apparently equally important needs
5. Must choose from several alternative ways of meeting needs

Nursing interventions are supportive, generative, or protective (see Chapter Two); they help the client or the family to meet their needs; they teach new and better ways of meeting needs; they correct faulty or inappropriate coping so that the client or the family can effectively meet needs. Quite often nurses help the client or the family identify health needs.

The ability to identify nursing problems rests on the accuracy and the completeness of the assessment. Among other things, the assessment points out the client's and the family's needs, their past responses to health problems, their present coping patterns and their degree of success in coping with the current health situation. A practical and useful way of identifying problems from the above information is to use the stress-response model presented in Chapter Two. The stress-response model hypothesizes that man responds to stress in an individual and holistic manner. This response is man's way of coping and his degree of coping success is evident in his ability to meet his needs. The stress-response model helps the nurse organize the assessment into a framework from which nursing problems can be extracted.

The major advantage to the stress-response model in planning care is that it determines the dynamics of the health situation. It not only identifies the general health problem and specifically the nursing problem, but it identifies the cause of the problem and the individual's ability to handle it. The nurse is therefore able to intervene more suitably, utilizing the client's own coping behavior to solve the problem. Unlike other approaches, the stress-response model does not place nursing care solely in the hands of the nurse. It determines the client's strengths and encourages the nurse to build nursing care that maximizes his potential.

The following examples demonstrate how the assessment and the stress-response model can be used to identify nursing problems.

Example 1.

> **Data:** Mrs. P is a 23-year-old woman. She is 3½-months pregnant. This is her first pregnancy and she is very happy and excited about the coming baby. She states she is "a little scared about the birth process and that she knows only what her friends have told her." She is eager to know all about pregnancy, labor and delivery, and infant care. She also states that she "hopes to be a good mother."
>
> **Assessment:** Mrs. P, a 23-year-old primipara, who states she is a little scared about the birth process, is eager to be a good mother and to learn about all the phases of pregnancy, childbirth, and infant care.
>
> **Stress:** Pregnancy (changes in body image, changes in role, changes in physiological functioning of the body during pregnancy, process of labor and delivery)
>
> **Responses:** Happiness about forthcoming birth. Eagerness to learn about pregnancy, birth process, and infant care. Fear about labor and delivery.
>
> **Unmet need:** Knowledge about labor and delivery, infant care, and pregnancy.
>
> **Problem(s):** How to design teaching concerning pregnancy, labor and delivery, and infant care for Mrs. P, considering her desire to learn and her fear about the birth process? How to help Mrs. P make the transition from nonmother role to mother role?

Note that the problems are stated clearly, specifically, and are goal-oriented; they have a built-in objective. The goal or objective of the first problem is to teach Mrs. P. The goal of the second problem is to help Mrs. P make the transition to mother role. The nursing interventions will determine *how* the goals are met.

Example 2.

> **Data:** Carolyn is a 6-year-old child. She is hospitalized in an acute stage of leukemia. She is weak and anorexic. She is receiving intravenous fluids but the physician is anxious to get her to take oral nourishment. Her gums bleed spontaneously, particularly when she eats abrasive foods. She requests toast for breakfast.
>
> **Assessment:** Carolyn, a weak and anorexic 6-year-old child in an acute stage of leukemia, who needs nourishment and whose gums bleed easily when she eats, desires toast for breakfast.

Stress: Proliferation of cells that destroy bone marrow, which reduces the production of erythrocytes and thrombocytes.

Responses: Poor nutrition, bleeding and anemia, poor appetite.

Unmet need: Nourishment during an acute stage of leukemia.

Problem: How to increase the leukemic child's nutritional status by utilizing her food preferences, when such food is liable to produce spontaneous bleeding from her gums?

In this example, the child's desire for toast creates the nursing problem. The nurse knows that toast is an abrasive food and by identifying the stress and the response it is obvious that if the nurse gives the child the toast, spontaneous bleeding may occur. Yet the nurse needs to include the child's food preferences in the plan of care, particularly when the child has a poor appetite as this child does. Use of the stress-response model and the assessment brings these points clearly into view and makes problem identification complete and accurate.

Example 3.

Data: Mr. S is hospitalized on an acute psychiatric unit. He is agitated, hostile, and often abusive. He paces continuously, talks incessantly, and has not eaten for days. His conversation is disjointed and incoherent. When he is visited by his family or friends he becomes more agitated. Two weeks ago his wife left him. Two days ago his business, a small electronics firm, collapsed in bankruptcy.

Assessment: Mr. S, a hyperactive, hostile, and extremely anxious man, who talks incessantly and incoherently, needs food to maintain adequate nutritional status.

Stress: Loss of wife two weeks ago, loss of business through bankruptcy.

Response: Increased anxiety manifested in manic behavior (hyperactivity, hyperverbalization, hostility, agitation, and incoherent conversation); not eating for days.

Unmet needs: Food and fluids. An appropriate way to cope with stress.

Problem(s):   How to get Mr. S to take food and fluids, when he is constantly moving about and talking incessantly? How to help Mr. S cope with his stress in a manner that does not interfere with his health?

In this example the nursing problem is evident in Mr. S's inability to appropriately handle his stress—the loss of his wife and his business. When the client is unable to gratify his needs for love and security and utilizes coping patterns that exclude food and fluid intake, health problems result. Problem identification in this case rests with the nurse's knowledge of man's basic needs for food and fluids and of the normal behavioral responses to stress.

The data indicate Mr. S's response is maladaptive, that is, it is creating further health problems for him. Mr. S needs food and fluids to maintain life processes and he needs to handle his stress more appropriately. Both of these unmet needs have been stated as nursing problems.

Example 4.

> **Data:** Laurie is a 15-year-old sophomore in high school. Her brother Timmy has cerebral palsy and is visited weekly by a public health nurse. During one of the visits, Laurie tells the nurse that she fainted last week. After questioning, the nurse refers Laurie to a physician. He diagnosed her problem as anemia and instructed the nurse to evaluate the family's dietary practices. After discussion with the mother, it was determined that everyone in the family ate well-balanced meals with the exception of Laurie. Laurie frequently dieted to maintain a slim size seven and was very concerned about remaining popular with the "crowd."
>
> **Assessment:** Laurie, a 15-year-old girl, who frequently diets to maintain a slim figure, has anemia caused by a dietary deficiency.
>
> **Stress:** Improper dieting during adolescence.
>
> **Response:** Anemia, size seven figure, fainting.
>
> **Unmet need:** A well-balanced diet for adolescent growth.
>
> **Problem:** How to help Laurie plan meals that provide needed nutrients for a well-balanced diet and that correct anemic problem and help her maintain slim size seven figure?

In this situation the nurse helped the family identify the health problem. Clues from Laurie prompted the nurse to refer her to a physician. Further gathering of data from the mother and the physician helped the nurse make the assessment. The unmet need becomes obvious when the stress and the response are identified. In this case the unmet need is the result of the stress.

Another example may help the reader to understand the use of the stress-response model for identifying nursing problems.

Example 5.

> **Data:** Mrs. D is the mother of four children. She was recently hospitalized in diabetic coma. She was diagnosed a diabetic after the birth of her last child. She is home now and with her children, aged 1 year, 3 years, 6 years, and 10 years. The public health nurse receives a call from Mr. D and he tells her that he is worried about the children, since he knows his wife is not taking her insulin and that she is "nipping" again. While talking to the husband the nurse learns that Mrs. D drinks wine, does not eat much, and is usually quite intoxicated by three o'clock in the afternoon. Mr. D knows that she forgets to feed the children and leaves them unattended as she sleeps in the bedroom. He has tried to get her to stop drinking but says that she cannot tolerate the thought of having to take a

shot every day and of having a disease like diabetes, so she drinks to "soothe her nerves."

Assessment: Mrs. D, a diabetic who has not accepted her health problem (diabetes) and who was recently hospitalized in diabetic coma, is drinking wine until she is intoxicated, is not eating properly or taking her daily insulin, and is not taking proper care of her four children.

Stress: Diabetes.

Response: Nonacceptance of diabetes with inappropriate means of handling nervousness (drinking wine); not properly caring for children.

Unmet needs: Acceptance of disease process (diabetes). Ability to cope with stress so as not to create more stress or complicate the diabetic state by drinking wine.

Problem(s): How to help Mrs. D accept her diabetic condition? How to help Mrs. D handle her feelings of "nervousness" so that she does not complicate the diabetic condition.

Problem identification in this example is seen in Mrs. D's maladaptive response to her diabetic condition. Mrs. D's response is her way of handling the stress of diabetes. Although her body is making efforts to cope with the metabolic imbalance, without the added insulin it is impossible for Mrs. D to maintain health. Mrs. D further complicates the health picture by drinking wine, which can trigger even more serious diabetic complications. It is evident from the analysis of the data coupled with an identification of the response that Mrs. D's unmet need is to accept her diabetic condition and to learn to handle her "nervousness" more appropriately. These needs then are the problems the nurse must help the client solve.

From these examples it seems clear that problem identification is the result of the nurse's ability to

1. Assess each situation accurately and completely
2. Supplement the assessment with knowledge from the behavioral and natural sciences
3. Place this information into a framework that helps organize, analyze, and identify the stress, the response, and the unmet need

With all of the preceding examples the nurse is required to identify the stress and the response in order to determine the nursing problem. Using this process of determining the nursing problem it is also necessary to decide whether the stress or the response is responsible for the unmet need. Either the stress is of such a nature or magnitude that the coping mechanisms cannot handle it or the individual's coping mechanisms are immature, inappropriate, or insufficient to handle the stress. In either case an unmet need develops. If there is no apparent way of meeting the unmet need, a problem exists.

Throughout the process of identifying a nursing problem, the nurse

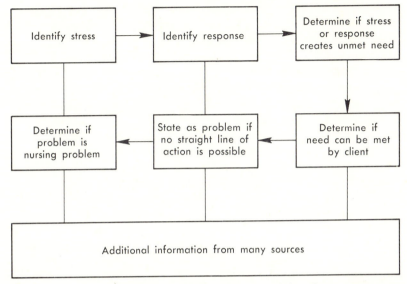

Fig. 5. Process of identifying nursing problems utilizing the stress-response model.

collects additional information. Data from observations, conversations, medical records, consultations, treatment plans, laboratory findings, and other paramedical personnel contribute to the ongoing assessment. This additional information enables the nurse to refine or revise the nursing problem. A schematic drawing of the steps in identifying a nursing problem utilizing the stress-response model is shown in Fig. 5.

As indicated in Fig. 5, problem identification utilizing the stress-response model is an open-ended process. At any stage in the process, refining and revision of the problem statement is possible. Additional information is sought throughout the process and is combined with nursing knowledge to formulate, predict, or revise present nursing problems or potential ones.

Criteria for stating the nursing problem

The ability to identify nursing problems and solve them is a major part of nursing activity. Problem statements need to be clear, simple, complete, and specific. They should reflect the problem situation so that the task of determining nursing approaches can be undertaken.

Problem statements are clear and simple. Problems need to be clearly, simply, and completely stated. Without a clear, unambiguous statement of the problem, the nurse cannot know what to solve or what decisions need to be made. A fundamental rule to keep in mind when stating a problem is: if you want to solve a problem, you must know what the problem is. It can be said that a large part of the solution of a problem lies in knowing what it is you are trying to do.

What is a good statement? Although there is no right way to state a problem, those problems that are stated in question form are simplest.[4] Question statements have the virtue of posing problems directly. Questions that begin with a "how" or "what" and that indicate the nursing objective, give direction. For example, "How to relieve Mrs. M's cough so that she can sleep at night?" tells the nurse what is to be accomplished by the nursing action. A question such as "What can be done for Mr. K to help him learn to manipulate the insulin syringe when his hands are crippled with arthritis?" clearly indicates the intent of the nursing plan.

Problem statements are specific. Problem statements that are specific give the nurse a goal. Statements that are general or too global do not give definite direction to the nurse for solution. The problem, "How to reduce the incidence of venereal disease in the community?" is so general a statement that the nurse needs to identify several subproblems before nursing action can be considered.

Since nursing problems arise when a person cannot meet his own needs, problem statements need to include a reference to the obstacle that blocks the person's ability to meet his needs. If the person has an unmet need but knows how to handle the situation, then no problem exists. Problems with a high degree of specificity include some reference to the obstacle that blocks the goal's attainment. An example might be: "How to prevent skin breakdown on Mr. J's buttocks when he must remain on his back in leg traction at all times?" In this statement the obstacle creating the problem is Mr. J's inability to move because of leg traction.

Nursing problems that are stated clearly, that are unambiguous, and that indicate the obstacle that is causing the problem provide the nurse with a definitive statement and an idea of how to approach a solution. Sometimes it is difficult to specifically identify the nursing problem in early contacts with the client. But as more data are collected a refining of the problem statement for specificity is desirable and often possible.

Problem statements communicate the nursing intent. To be meaningful, problem statements should communicate the nursing intent. When a problem statement includes a statement of the directional goal the nursing intent is known. Any member of the health team is then able to understand what it is the client needs and in what direction the nursing care is likely to be pointed. To state the nursing problem as "How to handle Mrs. F's anxiety?" does not convey the nursing intent. "How to reduce Mrs. F's preoperative anxiety

---

[4]Kerlinger, Fred N.: Foundations of behavioral research, New York, 1965, Holt, Rinehart & Winston, Inc., p. 19.

concerning her fear of inadequate postsurgical analgesia?" tells the nursing staff the source of Mrs. F's anxiety and that reduction of anxiety is the nursing goal. In the first statement, the words "to handle" do not specifically convey the nursing intent and therefore leave the problem statement in an ambiguous state. Problem statements that succinctly state the nursing intent also convey specificity. In other words, the statement of the client's problem identifies what is wrong while the statement of the nurse's problem states the nurse's *intent* in solving the problem. For instance:

Client's problem: Mrs. F is afraid of pain after surgery.

Nurse's problem: How to reduce Mrs. F's preoperative anxiety concerning her fear of postoperative pain?

Nursing problems that are simply stated in a question form, that are specific and communicate intent convey the goal of the nursing intervention. No nursing problem can be solved adequately without a clear and specific statement of the nursing problem.

In this chapter a framework for identifying nursing problems has been presented along with a discussion on assessment, problem identification, and the statement of the nursing problem. Chapter Four covers the next phase in the nursing process—planning for nursing action.

SUMMARY

The process of planning nursing care begins with an assessment and ends with assessment progressing through several phases. Assessment involves the collection, classification, and analysis of data to determine client or family needs and nursing problems. Data that describe the client's or the family's past experiences, practices, and reactions to health care are known as the nursing history. The nursing history and data concerning the client's present health needs are obtained from interviews, observations, medical records, and the literature.

Information gained from these many sources is then classified into groups with similar characteristics so that the nature, significance, and relationship of one group to another can be determined. Utilizing a deductive or an inductive analysis of these relationships, general statements about the client's or the family's health situation and the nursing implications are made to complete the assessment.

One way of determining nursing problems from the assessment is to use the stress-response model. The stress-response model enables the nurse to (1) identify the client's holistic response to stress; and (2) plan care that maximizes the client's or the family's present coping behaviors to solve the problem.

Suggested readings

Aguilera, Donna C., Messick, Janice M., and Farrell, Marlene S.: Crisis intervention, St. Louis, 1970, The C. V. Mosby Co., p. 57-117.

Burrill, Marjorie: Helping students identify and solve problems, Nurs. Outlook, February, 1966, pp. 46-48.

Campbell, Margaret: Identifying nursing problems, The Canad. Nurse, February, 1965.

Caplan, Gerald: An approach to community mental health, New York, 1961, Grune and Stratton, Inc., p. 33-63.

Fast, Julius: Body language, New York, 1970, J. B. Lippincott Co.

Folta, Jeannette, and Deck, Edith S., editors: A sociological framework for patient care, New York, 1966, John Wiley & Sons, Inc.

Fox, Madeline J.: Talking with patients who can't answer, Amer. J. Nurs. **71**(6):1146-1149, 1971.

Hardiman, Margaret A.: Interviewing or social chit-chat, Amer. J. Nurs. **71**(7):1379-1381, 1971.

Hewitt, Helen E., and Pesznecker, Betty L.: Blocks to communicating with patients, Amer. J. Nurs. **64**(7):101-103, 1964.

Johnson, Miriam M.: A sociological analysis of the nurse role. In Social interaction and patient care, Philadelphia, 1965, J. B. Lippincott Co., pp. 29-39.

Klagsbreen, Samuel C.: Communications in the treatment of cancer, Amer. J. Nurs. **71**(5):944-948, 1971.

Komorita, Nori I.: Nursing diagnosis, Amer. J. Nurs. **63**(12):83-86, 1963.

McCabe, Grace: Cultural influences on patient behavior, Amer. J. Nurs. **60**(8):1101-1104, 1960.

Parsons, Talcott: On becoming a person, The social system, New York, 1964, Free Press of Glencoe, pp. 436-443, 445-447.

Rae, Nancy Mara: Caring for patients following open heart surgery, Amer. J. Nurs. **63**(11):77-82, 1963.

Robischon, Paulette, and Scott, Diane: Role theory and its application in family nursing, Nurs. Outlook **17**(7):52-53, 1969.

Ruesch, Jurgen: The observer and the observed: human communication theory, Toward a unified theory of human behavior, New York, 1956, Basic Books, Inc., Publishers, pp. 36-54.

Stevens, Leonard F.: Nurse-patient discussion groups, Amer. J. Nurs. **63**(12):67-69, 1963.

Wesseling, Elizabeth: The adolescent facing amputation, Amer. J. Nurs. **65**(1):91-94, 1965.

Chapter

4

THE PROCESS OF SELECTING NURSING ACTIONS
AND FORMULATING EVALUATIVE CRITERIA

My own decision is . . . a human decision, made in freedom informed and governed by beliefs and values, as well as by attitudes and a fundamental perspective. It is a discernment of compassion . . . as well as of objective moral reflection. The judgment is made with a sense of its limitations, which include the limitations of the one who decides.

James F. Gustafson[1]

OVERVIEW

The formulation of a plan for action is the third phase of nursing care planning. It occurs after the assessment and identification of the client's needs and problems, yet it is definitely uppermost in the nurse's mind during the earlier phases. It requires both cognitive and testing behaviors. Studies of problem-solving behavior remind us that all persons do not go through the process of solving problems in exactly the same manner, but that an analysis of the steps of problem-solving points out the requirements of logically satisfactory problem-solving behavior.

To solve a nursing problem the nurse analyzes the problem situation and the goal in an attempt to hypothesize possible solutions. The nurse considers possible actions and their consequences in order to select the best action. This is known as the generative phase of problem solving; various resolutions or solutions to the problem are proposed and evaluated, using a variety of heuristic strategies to accomplish the task. Successful resolution of a problem requires that the nurse think through any number of possible solutions before a selection is made. This chapter (1) investigates the process of making a decision and presents a systematic method for the consideration of

[1]Gustafson, James F.: A Protestant ethical approach. In Noonan, John T., Jr. editor: The morality of abortion, Cambridge, 1971, Harvard University Press, p. 117.

alternatives and their consequences, and (2) presents an evaluative set of criteria for measuring the success of a selected nursing action.

There are several steps in planning for nursing action. At first they will seem involved, lengthy, and cumbersome, but any new behavior requires practice for the nurse to become skillful in its execution. Hopping back and forth between these steps is common to all problem solvers because we do not have the capacity to see the situation from every point of view at one time. But because we tend to view a problem in terms of its solution, it is useful to keep the goal in mind as solutions are considered.

GENERATING ALTERNATIVES

The process of making a decision about how to resolve a problem begins with the generation of possible solutions. Once the problem has been identified the nurse begins to consider solutions. Some are feasible, others are not. By analyzing the problem situation the nurse is able to sort out irrelevant solutions and to establish the action or actions most likely to solve the problem. During a critique of the problam situation the nurse is able to determine the type of problem. The identification of the type of problem directly affects the kind of alternatives the nurse can generate for solution. The nature of the problem influences the number, kind, and quality of the alternatives. Other things that influence the number, kind, and quality of alternatives are the data the nurse has gathered about the problem situation, the client, and the particular problem. If the goal for the nursing care is known and the nurse is able to identify what stands in the way of goal attainment, it is no time before solutions can be generated. Problems exist when goal attainment is thwarted by:

1. An interference or barrier to the achievement of the goal
2. No clearly established means of attaining the goal
3. Having to make a choice between two equally attractive goals, which creates conflict

If the problem is caused by a blocked goal, the nurse tries to determine how to remove the obstacle. The situation is examined for clues to determine what particular action will eliminate the interference and what tools will be needed to carry out the action. If the problem is one of blocked communication between the nurse and the client, the first step will be to identify what blocks the communication. The nurse may be skilled in opening the communicative lines or may need to get help via the literature or in consultation with experts in the field of communication.

When a problem exists because there is no clearly defined means of reaching the goal, the nurse initiates resolution by clearly identifying the goal. Once the goal is known, possible alternative approaches can be proposed. Problems of this kind almost always demand extensive data collection or help

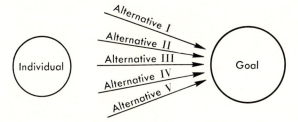

A problem exists when there is a goal to be attained, but the individual sees no well-defined, well-established means of attaining it, or when there are several alternative pathways to reaching the goal and the individual needs to choose the alternative which offers the best solution.

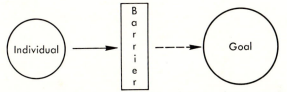

A problem exists when the individual is trying to reach a goal and a barrier interferes with goal attainment.

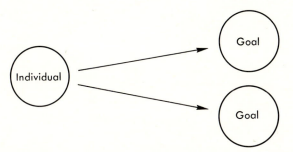

A problem exists when an individual must make a choice between two or more equally attractive goals. He finds himself in a conflict.

Fig. 6. Types of problem situations.

from resource people. If no means of goal attainment is evident it may mean the situation is not within the nurse's realm of experience or repertoire of knowledge. Frequently an outside source can provide the necessary data, expertise, and objectivity for resolution. Most often when adequate data are available several alternative solutions can be postulated.

Occasionally a problem occurs because the nurse has to make a decision between two equally desirable alternatives. When this happens the nurse must critically evaluate each alternative to determine which will provide the client with the best possible overall effect. The decision will include a consideration of the risk, value, and consequence of each alternative and of the availability of a means of meeting the goal. In most instances the decision is easier when it is analyzed in light of its total effect on the client's health. Consider for example this situation:

> Miss Layne, a community health nurse, had to decide whether to teach Mr. Klein, a newly diagnosed diabetic, self-care at home or refer him to a hospital for closer supervision. He had an intelligent and interested wife who had offered to help him learn self-care at home. However, Miss Layne knew he would receive excellent instruction at the hospital and would also be observed closely by highly qualified personnel.

This example presents a problem in which the nurse must decide between two alternatives toward one goal. The goal is to learn diabetic care. The two possible alternatives are: (1) teach Mr. Klein self-care at home with the help of his wife, or (2) refer him to the hospital for teaching with close supervision by qualified personnel. Some of the factors that may influence the choice of the action are:

1. The competency of the wife as a teacher
2. The motivation of the wife
3. The willingness of the husband to let the wife teach him
4. The cost of the hospitalization and the client's ability to handle the expense
5. The husband's previous experience with hospitalization

Each of these factors would be considered in light of its value and risk to the client and his wife before a choice could be made.

Unlike the problem situation presented above in which the nurse had to decide between two approaches toward one goal, occasionally problems arise when there are two goals with equally desirable end results but which are in opposition to one another. Suppose we alter the situation so that the decision rests between whether to teach Mr. Klein diabetic self-care or to continue to provide care.

> Mr. Klein is a newly diagnosed diabetic who says he wants to learn self-care but who exhibits fear about injections, disgust about testing urine, and is having some trouble staying on his new diet. Yet he is asking all about the disease process, and he wants to go home from the hospital very soon.

In this situation the nurse must decide between two conflicting alternatives to meet the goal. The goal is diabetic care. The two opposing alternatives are: (1) teach Mr. Klein self-care, or (2) provide care. Although Mr. Klein says he wants to learn self-care and go home, he is demonstrating many behaviors that make teaching difficult. Resolution of this conflict is influenced by many factors. Is Mr. Klein really ready for teaching? If not, what factors interfere with his readiness? If he has to stay in the hospital, will he eventually be able to learn, or would it be better to let him go home and have someone from a referring agency help? As the nurse raises these and many other questions, the dilemma begins to unfold, providing data for the generation of other alternatives. In any event the nurse must be able to identify the source of the problem and the nature of the problem before any alternative can be considered.

Now, let us change the situation so that there is no clearly established means of attaining the goal. For example:

> Mr. Klein is a 67-year-old, very independent blind man who is a newly diagnosed diabetic (extremely labile). He has ulcers on his feet, lives alone, is on welfare, and is becoming depressed while in the hospital. He states he misses his only companion, a big sheepdog named Fred. Miss Layne, the nurse, wants to get Mr. Klein home where he will be happier with his dog and to get him on a self-care regimen.

This situation offers a great deal of challenge. The goal again is self-care. The alternative means of meeting the goal are vague because of so many factors. But it is clear that the goal must be met and soon or Mr. Klein will have an additional problem. So the nurse begins to generate possible alternatives. He could go home and have a nurse visit each day to dress his ulcers, check his urine and diet, and give him the insulin; but that would interfere with Mr. Klein's independence. He could have a home health aide from the public health department come in and fix his meals and feed him, but again, that would impinge on the client's independence. Again and again, possible alternative actions are considered and their consequences evaluated until the nurse finds a solution that has a high probability of occurrence, a high value to the client, and a low risk to his health. Problems of this type tax the imaginative power of the nurse as possible solutions are raised. Such heuristic devices as brainstorming, guessing, fantasizing, purging, exploring, focusing, and searching,[2] to name a few, are used as the problem solver considers possible alternatives to solve the problem.

Finally, let us imagine Mr. Klein's problem is caused by a blocked goal. For example:

> Mr. Klein, a 67-year-old man recently diagnosed a diabetic, is refusing to learn how to give his own insulin. In fact, he refuses to let anyone give him the insulin, stating that he wants to take a pill. Although the physician has explained that a pill would not be possible since he needs insulin, he continues to refuse the injection.

[2]Straus, David and others: Tools for change, San Francisco, 1971, Interaction Associates, pp. 54-60.

The short-term goal in this situation is to get Mr. Klein to take his insulin injection. The long-term goal is to teach Mr. Klein to administer his own insulin injection. The barrier to immediate goal attainment is Mr. Klein's refusal to take the insulin injection. Many questions come to mind as the nurse assesses this situation. What is the reason Mr. Klein refuses the insulin injection? Is it fear, pain, or other feelings resulting from previous experience with injections? Does he understand the need for insulin in diabetic conditions like his? Does he understand the seriousness of the condition when the medication is not administered? Perhaps answers to these questions will enable the nurse to generate alternative actions, for Mr. Klein's refusal to take his medication is clearly a barrier to optimal health and is a risk to his well-being.

Hypothesizing: a heuristic device for generating alternatives

In any given problem situation the problem solver initially begins to consider solutions after he has analyzed the goal and determined what blocks goal attainment. He may hypothesize or tentatively assume that certain actions will remove the block. Some of his hypotheses are wild guesses, others are based on past experiences or on knowledge. One means of organizing needed information and theoretical knowledge for the purpose of determining actions is to use predictive principles. As stated by Douglas and Bevis in *Team Leadership in Action,* "organizing ideas and facts into [predictive] principles enables the nurse-leader to have a clear, categorized fund of knowledge for immediate use in nursing situations."[3] Principles are guides for developing realistic alternatives of action. Predictive principles are action hypotheses. They tell you what will promote or inhibit progress toward a desired goal. They provide the nurse with direction and they predict outcomes. By definition, "predictive principles are a set of circumstances, conditions, or behaviors that produce a given definable outcome.[4] Predictive principles express a relationship between the circumstances, conditions, and behaviors with the definable outcome. They describe what is going to happen as a result of the activation of the conditions, circumstances, or behaviors. They predict what the outcome of the relationship will be. In order for a predictive principle to be predictive it must be valid and be in active language, that is, have an active verb. An example of a predictive principle is: using predictive principles as a guide for nursing action provides the nurse with direction in making decisions about nursing actions. Predictive principles are a mechanism for determining what will be the possible consequences of proposed actions and what the value or risk will be.

---

[3]Douglas, Laura Mae, and Bevis, Em Olivia: Team leadership in action, St. Louis, 1970, The C. V. Mosby Co., p. 9.
[4]Douglas and Bevis: Team leadership in action, p. 3.

Hypotheses need to be tested in order to determine their ability to meet the required intent, that is, to remove the block to goal attainment. Since predictive principles are action hypotheses, their natural outcome is any number of activities that could be utilized to meet the predicted outcome. An example will illustrate this point. Suppose the predictive principle states: complete and accurate data collection increases the probability of accurate problem identification. From this principle the nurse would consider all the actions possible for obtaining an accurate and complete collection of data. Data collection can be achieved in a variety of ways depending on the persons involved and the circumstances of the situation. A few alternative actions for collecting complete data, as discussed in Chapter Three, would be:

1. Observation
2. Interviewing
3. Consultation with other health professionals involved in the health situation
4. Review of the health records
5. Review of the literature related to the situation

The nurse may decide to carry out one action or to use all five in an attempt to collect complete data. To determine if the data are accurate, the nurse would need to do one or all of the following actions:

1. Analyze the data
2. Sort and classify the data
3. Check other resources for validation of the data

As the nurse identifies the alternative actions that would activate the principle it becomes evident that choices need to be made. Decisions concerning which action to use, when to act, and who is to act need to be made. A process for making a decision is needed.

PROCESS OF MAKING A DECISION

Since decision making is a complex behavior that requires the selection of a choice from many choices, it demands that the problem solver be able to analyze and select choices and organize them in order of the most desirable to the least desirable. The person who explores, brainstorms, or hypothesizes alternatives before making a decision is in a "learning stage"; he still wants to learn new and better ways of reaching his goal. There are several factors that influence the number of alternatives that can be considered before a decision is made. They are:

1. The number of alternatives the problem solver can weigh at one time before he becomes confused
2. The number of people who are participating and their problem-solving abilities
3. The amount of time available

If the nurse problem solver tries to dredge up every possible alternative, she may only end up confusing herself and wasting precious time in the process, for the nurse can actually consider only those alternatives that are known or seem possible. Research has found that executives weigh only two, three, or four alternatives when making a decision.[5] To go beyond this number confuses the mind because there are too many ideas to be analyzed.

When more than one person is making the choice of alternatives, the number of persons and their problem-solving skill determine how successful the venture will be. Group work becomes necessary when the decision directly affects the members of the group or when cooperation from the group members is needed. The greatest value of group decisions is that the group members have a chance to share, explore, and search for possible alternatives. What one member cannot discover, another can. Group decisions also have the advantage of shared responsibility for the decision. The disadvantage of group decisions is that they tend to take a longer time than a decision made by one person would take.

The nurse problem solver cannot spend too much time in exploring alternatives, or the decision will be made, for no matter how much time is available decisions *are* made. It is a rare problem situation that can stand too long without resolution. One way to learn when to stop considering alternatives is to exercise the decision after exploring a few alternatives and then evaluate the result. There are some problem situations that will be repeated, at which time the nurse can consider different or more alternatives. In this way the nurse can compare and contrast one situation with the other to improve the ability to propose possible alternative actions.

Consequences of alternatives

Before the nurse can decide on a choice or an alternative there must be a way to compare one alternative with another in order to select the best one. When the nurse considers the consequences of each alternative, the effects of the proposed action are studied. For every alternative there are usually several consequences. If a particular alternative is carried to completion a set of consequences or conclusions is possible. The consequences can be predicted with some assurance because any act can or cannot produce the desired effect.

Recall the predictive principle about data collection. The nurse had the choice of observing, interviewing, referring to resources, or reviewing the records for data. One of the consequences of observing the situation is that the nurse may gather valuable information, may get a little information, or may get none at all. Each particular situation will determine the result. But in any case the nurse can predict at least three distinct, possible consequences

---

[5] Forum, Fall-Winter ed., 1971, J. C. Penney Co.

for the action of observing. Other consequences are possible depending on the incident. More experienced nurses can predict with greater awareness, but even the novice can predict consequences with a high degree of accuracy if she thinks through all the possible results of any given act. The first criterion, then, for measuring the value of an alternative is to formulate *all* possible consequences so that they can be submitted for further evaluation.

Estimates of probability

Once the consequences of each alternative have been determined, it is necessary to estimate the likelihood of their occurrence. Although each alternative has several consequences, some are more likely to occur than others. This is known as their probability of appearance. Probability is defined as "the likelihood of the occurrence of an event, estimated as a ratio between the number of ways in which the event may occur and the number of ways in which alternative events may occur."[6] It is important to consider the probability of the consequences occurring when making a decision, because if the consequence is likely to occur very seldom the alternative has less weight when compared with an alternative with consequences of higher probability of occurrence. Probability is used when there is a need to know whether certain things will happen or not.

Probability is a *predicted* estimate of the event's occurrence. The estimate is based on past experience and on data pertinent to the situation. Imagine a situation in which the nurse is on duty on a labor and delivery unit in a large community hospital. The phone rings and is answered. A voice in an excited manner says, "I am Linda Richards. I am pregnant and I think I am in labor. This is my first baby and I'm not sure. What should I do?" The nurse immediately knows that more data are needed before she can tell Mrs. Richards what to do. In this incident, data could be collected in several ways. The nurse knows that many of the patients who deliver in this hospital are clinic patients and therefore have medical records that can be checked. Data can also be collected from the patient. Certainly her physician could give needed information. So the nurse has at least three sources from which to collect data. Let us look at the consequences of each choice, and the probability of occurrence of each consequence.

From Fig. 7, the nurse would most likely select Actions 1 and 2 in order to get a complete compilation of data. Consequence (a) of Action 1 gives the nurse information about the present situation, and Consequence (a) of Action 2 gives the nurse information about the client's prenatal period. Both have a high probability of occurrence and together provide the desired information. Consequence (b) of Action 1 has a low probability of occurrence and is

---

[6]Merriam-Webster, A.: Webster's Third New International Dictionary, Vol. II, Chicago, 1966, William Benton, Publisher, p. 1806.

ACTION	CONSEQUENCES	PROBABILITY OF OCCURENCE
1. Interview Mrs. Richards	(a) will find out what is happening right now	high
	(b) will not find out what is happening right now	low
	(c) will find out about the prenatal period	medium
	(d) will not find out about the prenatal period	medium
2. Send for her record	(a) will get record with information	high
	(b) will not get record	low
	(c) will not get information about immediate situation	high
3. Call her doctor	(a) will be able to reach him and get needed information	medium
	(b) will reach him and not be able to get needed information	low
	(c) will not be able to reach him	medium

Fig. 7. Consequences and their probabilities.

therefore negated by Consequence (a), since they are two sides of the same coin—when one is highly probable, the other is highly improbable. The same is true of Consequences (a) and (b) of Action 2. Consequences (d) of Action 1 and (c) of Action 2 reciprocate each other when both actions are carried to completion. Action 3, however, can be ruled out because all the consequences have a low to medium probability of occurrence. Analysis of Action 3 reveals it is not an approach that will yield the desired information; it is unlikely the action, if carried to completion, will produce the needed information.

This example points out the value of using a probability measure to determine choices of alternatives. If the event's consequences seldom occur, they have less weight, when compared with consequences that occur more often. If the consequence occurs a high percentage of the time, it most likely will negate the other consequences' occurrence. It is important to remember that probability is used to estimate the occurrence of the *consequence* of an alternative, and not the occurrence of the alternative itself.

In order to evaluate the probable occurrence of the consequence of an event, the relative frequency of that consequence must be determined and compared with the frequency of other consequences. Numbers representing degrees of probability may be used to symbolize this estimate. If this estimated consequence occurs with great frequency, that is, nine times out of ten, it receives a numerical value of 0.90. If the occurrence has a low incidence of appearance, say one or two times out to ten, it receives a low numerical rating of 0.10 or 0.20. Decimals or fractions can be used to designate the frequency of occurrence. Multiples of ten are used for simplicity: 0.10 or 1/10 means one out of ten times the event will occur; 0.90 or 9/10 means the event occurs nine out of ten times. Sometimes percentage is used: 0.90 or 9/10 is the same as 90%; 0.10 or 1/10 is the same as 10%. Numerical ratings are an excellent way of rating a consequence's occurrence because they convey levels or grades of probability. A high probability of occurrence is rated as 0.99 to 0.80; a probable occurrence is 0.79 to 0.60; a questionable occurrence is 0.59 to 0.50; a low probability occurrence is 0.49 to 0.30; and a very low probability occurrence is 0.29 to 0.10.

An alternative method for expressing probability estimates is to state them as high, medium, or low. For example, an event that occurs as often as seven or more times out of ten is considered to have a high probability of occurrence; whereas a consequence that only occurs one or two times out of ten has a low probability of occurrence. If the event has a frequency of five out of ten times it demonstrates a medium occurrence. As with the numerical estimates, words like high, medium, and low convey a relative frequency of occurrence as measured by the number of times an event occurs out of ten times. Estimates of probability that are expressed by words look like this:

High probability occurrence = Seven or more times out of ten

Medium probability occurrence = Four to six times out of ten

Low probability occurrence = One to three times out of ten

The probability of an occurrence of a consequence is based on objective and subjective estimates.[7] *Objective estimates* are the result of the systematic recording of the frequency with which different consequences occur. *Subjective estimates* are based on the nurse's own memory of the frequency of an occurrence as reported by other nurses or experienced by herself. Emotional factors often influence the nurse's estimates. If the nurse has had a traumatic experience with an alternative, the memory is likely to affect the estimate of its occurrence. The nurse is likely to remember the consequence as unpleasant, causing her to overestimate the likelihood of the occurrence.

---

[7]Bailey, June T., MacDonald, Frederick J., and Claus, Karen E.: An experiment in nursing curriculums at a university. Unpublished terminal report of the experimental curriculum evaluation project, School of Nursing, University of California at San Francisco, 1971, p. 48.

Subjective estimates are often extrapolations of theory or of inference made from data collected about the situation.

At this time in the development of nursing, exact numerical values cannot be stated. However, a scale of *estimated values* is a useful tool for communicating probability of occurrence. The main point to be remembered when using numerical values is that the numbers only communicate an idea to all of those using them.

Desirability of consequence

Obviously the choice between alternatives is not solely dependent on the likelihood of a consequence occurring. If that were so, the nurse would simply choose the alternative that is most likely to occur. The value of the consequence also needs to be considered, for a highly likely occurrence may be highly undesirable and a highly improbable occurrence may be highly desirable. Since any one alternative usually has more than one consequence, each must be evaluated for its desirability. The consequence would be desirable if it (1) accomplished the preferred intent, (2) did not have any harmful or troublesome side effects or after effects, and (3) is the most efficient and appropriate way to meet the preferred goal. The value or desirability of a consequence can be represented arbitrarily by a positive or a negative symbol.

One way in which the nurse problem solver can determine the desirability of a consequence is by evaluating its risk to the client. If the consequence has harmful side effects or after effects, it must be carefully evaluated before use. If the consequence has questionable or temporary results, it may also be risky in that it does not necessarily accomplish the preferred intent. Some highly probable consequences have serious side effects and are therefore not desirable. Although freedom from pain is desirable, when the client has a sensitivity to a certain analgesic, the result of using that analgesic would make it undesirable. Another analgesic would have to be used instead. Some nursing actions, though, are used regardless of the risk because not to act in such a manner would be riskier than to act. It is risky to get a unilateral amputee up for the first time to walk with crutches because he may fall, but not to get him up is riskier in that he may begin to believe he is not able to manage crutches. The nurse decides the risk of falling is not such a great threat that she will not let the client try. She chooses to risk a fall rather than risk the chance that the client will lose faith in his ability to manage with crutches. It is always better to take a course of action that leads to the maximization of the client's potential. Precautions can be used to minimize the risk involved. Fig. 8 illustrates a decision-making schema for analyzing a nursing alternative by evaluating the probability, value, and risk of a consequence.

There are several guidelines for helping the nurse make a decision:

Guideline one. Choose the alternative that leads to as many desirable

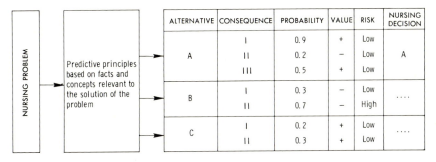

Fig. 8. Decision-making schema.

consequences as possible. This means the nurse must consider the consequences of each alternative in light of their threat to life, integrity, and safety to the client, the nurse, and other members of the health team. The nurse must ask "do the predicted consequences of this alternative meet the desired goal?" "Will the alternative have a temporary or long-term effect?" "Does the alternative create a risk?" "Does the risk result from a consequence that has a low probability of occurrence and, if so, do the other consequences of that alternative outweigh that risk?" Ideally, the selected alternative should have the most desirable consequences.

Guideline two. Select the alternative that best meets the desired intent but that minimizes risk to all involved. There are times when it is not possible to choose an alternative that does not have a risk. The safest strategy would be to choose the alternative that has the greatest potential for success yet the least degree of risk. When faced with a decision between one or more alternatives that have undesirable consequences, the least risky is the one that has the lowest probability of occurrence. Probability, in this instance, is the factor that determines the choice.

Guideline three. When faced with a decision between risk to the client or risk to an agency, the nurse, or other health team members, prime consideration goes to the client. The client, by virtue of his need for help, deserves first consideration. Compromise action may be necessary if the risk to others is also high. Fortunately, there are not too many instances when decisions of this sort are required. Most often they occur during life-threatening situations in which the nurse may initiate an action that poses a risk to her licensure. In such case, the risk to licensure must be weighed against the threat to the client's life, and the decision must be made accordingly.

Guidelines such as the above provide the nurse with a means for making nursing decisions. Some decisions do not, when carried to completion, meet the desired goal. When this happens the nurse will reassess the situation by conceptualizing the alternatives available and will then make a second decision using the same guidelines.

The advantage of conceptualizing alternatives and their consequences before actualization is that it calls attention to what may occur and allows the nurse to choose the seemingly best approach. It cuts down on trial-and-error approaches and on rigidity of response. It does not necessarily guarantee that the best approach will be reached. If anything, decisions that are based on an analysis of the alternatives allow the nurse to reconstruct the nursing actions and the steps of problem solution as hypotheses for testing. Having reconstructed the actions, the nurse can then implement or test the hypotheses and evaluate the total process. Many nurses revise their nursing plans as they enact them and observe the consequences of the enactments. Nurses who have learned to deliberately and consciously consider the alternatives available to them during the planning phase not only save time and energy, but more importantly they also are more apt to meet the client's needs more efficiently.

The following example of a depressed client illustrates the foregoing discussion of the decision-making process:

Data: Mr. Fox is a 55-year-old man who has been admitted to the psychiatric unit in severe depression. He is an unemployed electrical engineer who has been out of work for 9 months. He was admitted last night because his wife is unable to tend him. Over the last 2 months he has become increasingly depressed until he has not eaten or slept for the last 4 days. His wife is unable to get him to care for himself, to eat or take fluids, or to handle his bowel or bladder needs. Last night he did not sleep and he needed to be routed out of bed this morning and dressed. He refused to eat breakfast even though the psychiatric technician tried to feed him in the dining room. He is now sitting in the dayroom with his head down. He is unkempt, unshaven, and motionless. Beneath his chair is a puddle of urine. Although there is much activity in the room, Mr. Fox seems not to be aware of all the noise, since he neither blinks nor lifts his head.

Assessment: Mr. Fox is severely depressed and needs food and fluids, and to maintain the daily acts of living (sleep, mobility, dressing, bowel and bladder care).

Stress: Loss of job.

Response: Loss of interest in the acts of daily living. Loss of interest in eating. Inability to sleep. Immobility. Depression (loss of self-worth, self-esteem, and self-respect) manifested in extreme melancholy.

Problem(s): How to increase Mr. Fox's sense of self-esteem, self-respect, and self-worth?

NURSING PROBLEM	PREDICTIVE PRINCIPLES (guides to action)	ALTERNATIVES	CONSEQUENCES	PROBABILITY	VALUE	RISK	NURSING DECISION
How to increase Mr. Fox's sense of self-esteem, self-respect and self-worth.	• The level of depression determines the type of nursing action.	1. Sit next to Mr. Fox and try to get him to verbalize his feelings.	He will verbalize his feelings.	0.2	+	Low	......
	• An open and accepting attitude facilitates a development of trust.		He will not verbalize his feelings.	0.8	−	High	
How to get Mr. Fox to take fluids and food.	• The outward expression of aggression and hostile feelings decreases the possibility that these feelings will be turned inward on oneself and thus lower one's sense of self-esteem.	2. Say, "You must feel very uncomfortable in those wet clothes, come with me and let's get you more comfortable". Get a male nurse or orderly if necessary.	He will know you care.	0.8	+	Low	Alternative 2
			He will feel cleaner.	0.9	+	Low	
			His dignity will have been preserved.	0.9	+	Low	
			His skin will be clean and less liable to break-down.	0.8	+	Low	
	• Believing someone cares promotes feelings of worth.	3. In the privacy of his room, offer Mr. Fox sips of fruit juice and selections of food.	He will take juice and food.	0.7	+	Low	Alternative 3
	• Nursing interventions which are designed to encourage severely depressed persons toward acts of daily care protects that person from further deterioration.		He will not take juice and food.	0.3	−	Moderate	
	• Feelings of self-esteem, self-respect and acceptance enhance a positive and realistic self-concept, thus lifting feelings of depression.		His dignity and self-respect will be preserved since he has privacy.	0.8	+	Low	

Fig. 9. Decision-making sequence.

How to get Mr. Fox to:
  A. Take fluids and food
  B. Move about
  C. Handle his bowel and bladder needs
  D. Sleep

Fig. 9 demonstrates the decision-making sequence of the first problem: how to increase Mr. Fox's sense of self-esteem, self-respect, and self-worth? A similar process would be necessary to plan for Problem 2.

In some cases the selection of alternatives is not an either/or decision, but would include several of the alternatives proposed. As shown in Fig. 9, the selection of Approaches 2 and 3 would be made because they together achieve the optimum results in solving the nursing problem. The analyzed decisions seem to logically follow Guidelines 1 and 2; that is, they take courses of action that lead to as many desirable consequences as possible and avoid a course of action that may lead to a highly undesirable consequence. Action 1 has an undesirable consequence with a probability of occurrence of 0.8; whereas Action 2 has four consequences that are all highly desirable and highly probable. Action 3 has one consequence that is highly probable and highly desirable and one alternative that is moderately probable and highly desirable. The main reason that Action 1 has a highly improbable and highly undesirable consequence is that it presupposes a severely depressed person can verbalize his feelings. The probability of this occurrence is very low and is therefore very undesirable. Knowledge of the psychodynamics of depression enables the nurse to estimate the low probability of this consequence.

Actions for Mr. Fox's level of depression should be directed toward helping him feel better about himself. An improved appearance will improve his sense of worth because his sense of worth is deeply affected by how he sees himself. Since Mr. Fox does not have the energy to tend to his own needs, he will need to be cleaned up, his clothes will need to be changed, and his skin will need to be cleansed. But the way in which he is cleansed is important, since it will affect his sense of dignity. Having a male nurse rather than a female nurse perform this action is one way of preserving his sense of dignity. Feeding him in private rather than in the dining room is another way. Few things are more deflating to the ego than having wet pants changed or having to be fed. Both activities, if not carefully and tastefully carried out, can create a feeling of low self-esteem. The consequences with their probabilities, risk, and value of Alternatives 2 and 3 demonstrate the above points.

As Mr. Fox begins to regain his sense of self-worth and dignity he will begin to feel better about himself, and his depression will begin to lift. As the depression lifts he will again have the energy to become involved in self-care and be able to verbalize his feelings.

To develop approaches that are creative and individualized requires the sort of critical analysis outlined above. Only then will clients be assured of care that is deliberately customized to meet their needs.

PRIORITY SETTING FOR SELECTED NURSING ACTIONS

Ranking nursing actions in their order of priority will:

1. Provide for the most efficient, the safest, and the quickest means of meeting a desired goal
2. Separate actions for meeting short-term goals from actions to meet long-term goals
3. Determine which action comes first for maximum therapeutic effect

When there is more than one action to meet the desired goal, it becomes necessary that the actions be carried out in such a way that the desired goal is met in the quickest and most efficient manner possible. Therefore some actions take precedence over others. For example, quick reduction of an elevated temperature in a child with possible pneumonia takes precedence over sending him to the x-ray unit for a chest film. A reverse order of actions could be harmful for the child.

Nursing actions are considered when setting priorities, and the nurse takes into consideration the possibility that the consequence of one action might contribute to the attainment of another goal. For example, the demonstrated interest and concern of the nurse who is administering to the physical needs of the client goes a long way toward helping the client feel worthy and accepted.

Separating actions that meet long-term goals from actions that meet short-term goals is a natural sequela for determining which actions are feasible. For instance, if the goal of the nursing care is to help the client accept his dependency needs, then the action of listening and helping the client sort out his feelings comes before any action that helps him cope with his feelings. The action that meets the immediate goal is designed to help the client identify his fears and fantasies concerning his dependency. Actions that meet the long-term goal help the client accept the dependency feelings by developing ways in which he can experience dependency in a positive and rewarding manner.

Sometimes priority setting of nursing actions is determined by the desired therapeutic effect. When the desired therapeutic effect is to prevent pulmonary stasis, the alternatives for nursing action are as follows:

Action 1. Encourage the client to cough

Action 2 Percussion and vibration of the anterior and posterior chest to loosen secretions

Action 3. Endotracheal stimulation and suction as necessary

Priority order would place Action 2 over Action 1, followed by Action 3. The nurse would percuss and vibrate the client's chest to loosen secretions. Then, using either external mechanical tracheal stimulation or internal mechanical stimulation (resulting from prolonged exhalation), the client would be encouraged to cough. If these two mechanical attempts to stimulate a cough fail, then the nurse could introduce a nasal catheter to stimulate the trachea. The rationale for this priority ordering is as follows:

1. Percussion and vibration of the client's chest loosens secretions.
2. Most people, unless they are extremely debilitated, can cough up sputum into the pharynx and then expectorate it.
3. A catheter introduced into the trachea produces coughing.
4. Whenever a catheter is introduced into the trachea there is the possibility of having to use suction.
5. Tracheal suctioning can create multiple premature ventricular contractions, which can lead to cardiac arrest.

Therefore, the order of Action 2 followed by Actions 1 and 3 is necessary if the maximum therapeutic effect is to be accomplished with the lowest risk to the client.

In crisis situations in which life is threatened, the priority choice is the one that will have the greatest probability of saving the life. The person with a myocardial infarction is in severe pain, and if the pain is not relieved he may go into shock and die. It would seem, then, that the administration of pain medication would be the first nursing action. But when the nurse considers the source of the pain, the administration of oxygen takes precedence, since the pain is the result of a lack of oxygen to the heart muscle. Timing is a crucial factor in this situation. If the nurse chooses to administer the pain medication before the oxygen, the heart suffers a serious decrease of oxygen while the medication is being prepared and administered. In this case, a time lag could mean irreparable damage to the heart muscle.

The order of priority that the nurse establishes is influenced by several factors, such as (1) time, (2) external constraints (policies and legal statutes), (3) internal constraints (nurse's own values), and (4) how willing the nurse is to accept the external and internal constraints. Many nursing activities are independent of the physician's orders, but many are not. Priority setting is greatly influenced by the nurse's acceptance of the constraints of policy and the law when faced with situations that she deems in violation of these constraints. For instance, if a client is in a life-threatening situation and a physician is not accessible, the nurse will examine the situation, considering her own values, the law, and the policy of the agency. Intensive care and cardiac care units, emergency rooms, and outpatient clinics have standing orders for this very reason. How the nurse copes with the decision depends on how she accepts the risk involved if the action violates policy.

PLANS FOR EVALUATION

As the nurse plans for approaches to the delivery of nursing care, it becomes evident that some means of evaluating the care is also necessary. The fourth and final phase of nursing care planning is devoted to the creation of the evaluation plan. If nursing actions are designed to help the client meet a need or solve a problem, then the expected outcome of a nursing action describes how the client will look, feel, or be after the nursing action has been implemented. Once the nursing action has been selected and deemed the best approach to meet the need or to solve the problem, a means of evaluating the action is necessary. Many criteria for evaluation have been proposed for judging nursing behaviors. Isobel Stewart first developed guidelines in 1919 to standardize nursing procedures.[8] Since that time her guidelines have been modified for use in evaluating nursing personnel. Her criteria remain a useful tool and are good guidelines for measuring quality of care today.

As the nurse formulates these evaluative measures it is essential that she remember there are long-term goals and short-term expectations. The achievement of long-term goals cannot always be measured immediately. Plans are instituted to measure the immediate responses and then the long-term responses. When the nurse teaches the client about ways to remain free from illness, the short-term goal is that the client grasp the intent, the concepts, and the impact of the information. Some immediate change in behavior will be expected. The long-term expectation is that the knowledge will keep the client healthy and move him toward high-level wellness.

Criteria for evaluation

When planning evaluation criteria for nursing actions, it is important to include a precise description of the expected outcome. The terminal expectation of the nursing action should be described in unambiguous terms so that all those concerned will know what to expect. Mager's criteria for writing an objective is a good guideline to follow for clearly stating the expected outcome of a nursing action. He suggests that the terminal expectation be described by:

1. Identifying the specific behavior that will be accepted as evidence of the desired outcome
2. Defining the important conditions under which the behavior is to occur
3. Defining the criterion of acceptable performance[9]

A written criterion for the expected outcomes of a nursing action, then, states what changes will be evident in the client, the family, or the community as a result of the nursing action. If the nursing action is directed toward helping the client or his family, the terminal expectation must be stated in behavioral or performance terms. Behavior in this sense is used broadly to mean the physiological, psychological, social, and intellectual

---

[8]Stewart, Isobel M.: Possibilities of standardization in nursing techniques, Mod. Hosp., June 1919.

[9]Mager, Robert: Preparing instructional objectives, Belmont, 1962, Fearon Publishers, p. 53.

activities, as well as the observable responses. This would include not only those behaviors that can be observed but also all the data available that measure the less obvious responses. Such things as laboratory tests, x-rays, sociometric and psychological tests can be used as means of stating expected outcomes.

Nurses have multiple ways of determining outcomes and should use them more freely, since they most effectively provide objective evidence of behavior change. For example: Mrs. Smith demonstrates a normal tempera-ture when her thermometer reading registers between 98° and 99° F. Too often nurses identify outcomes in a subjective way. They use terms such as understand, enjoy, accept, promote, and maintain to explain expectation. But these terms do not clearly communicate the behavior. A laboratory test result, such as a white blood count of 7,000, conveys a normal white count. Each nurse who sees this will get the same idea. The same is true of observable behavior. Statements that clearly communicate what is seen and heard do not leave it up to the evaluator to figure out what to look for when the client "understands." Anything that can be observed or heard, such as a change in facial expression, posture, or tone of voice needs to be included, since these responses can convey whether an action is effective or not. If the client states he is in pain and cannot move his arm because of the pain, the evaluation criterion explicitly states how he will look and feel when the pain is gone: Mr. Jones will be free of pain when he is able to freely move his affected arm and when he states the pain is gone.

Sometimes the expected outcome of the nursing action will be written in light of the changes expected in the environment or the community. Environmental changes, program implementation, or any variety of other expectations can be included. Each statement describes what change is expected and how the change will look as a result of the nursing action. If the nursing action is to clean polluted water, then the expected color, clarity, and consistency of the water should be stated.

According to Mager's second point, in order to further clarify the expected terminal outcome of a nursing action, it will be necessary to state the condition under which the outcome will occur. Certain restrictions, situations, or requirements are necessary to completely define the terminal outcome. These conditions may be factors in the environment that alter the client's performance in some way, or they might be factors that describe how the client will perform. For example, while walking, the lower edge of Mr. Klein's cast will not rub an abrasive area on the top of his foot. The condition in this example is the walking, since this is the time when Mr. Klein's cast may rub his foot. Including the condition helps clearly define when the desired effect is to be expected. For example, Mr. Klein will walk to the solarium from his hospital room without assistance. In this example, the condition imposed on Mr. Klein's performance is that he will walk without assistance. The terminal act of walking to the solarium must be accomplished without aid. When the conditions for performance are included in the evaluative criteria, there is less chance for misunderstanding. Some behavioral acts can be misconstrued and therefore do not communicate the expected outcome. The clearer the criteria can be stated, the less chance there is for error or ambiguity.

Sometimes the conditions of the evaluative statement include "givens"; sometimes they have limitations or "restrictions." Often both are needed to clearly describe the expected outcome.

Example 1.
Given the necessary equipment, Mr. Klein will bathe himself.

The condition imposed on Mr. Klein in this statement is a "given." He will receive certain things that he will need for bathing himself.

Example 2.
Mr. Klein will bathe himself in bed.

The condition in this statement is a "restriction." He will bathe himself but it must be while he is in bed.

Example 3.
Given the necessary equipment, Mr. Klein will bathe himself while in bed.

Now the evaluative statement has both a "given" and a "restriction." Together they spell out the exact behavior that is expected. What it does not tell is how he will look after he has bathed. For that expected outcome another evaluative statement will be written.

A very frequent and important limitation is time. With rising costs in medical and nursing care, it is necessary to accomplish the most in the least amount of time. Time limitations also provide a clear delineation for measuring progress. Certain behaviors are expected at certain times; otherwise, a problem is indicated. For example, by the end of the second postoperative day, Mr. F, who had an appendectomy, will be free of nausea and vomiting. Expected outcomes that describe what to expect on the second day for this client must be realistic and within normal limits for the particular surgical procedure. If the client continues to vomit beyond the second day, it can be supposed that he has another problem. Time limits can also help measure the sequential steps in the completion of a long-term plan of care. In planning for the diabetic, the requirements and limitations that help determine progress need to be stated. In the early stages of teaching the client about diabetic self-care, an expected outcome might be: after practicing each day for a week, Miss J will be able to administer, without help, her own insulin injection; or, during hospitalization, Miss J will correctly test and interpret her daily urine sugar content; and, before going home, Miss J will be able to plan a meal that meets the caloric, protein, and fat allowances of her diabetic diet.

Since the above expected outcomes involve time and energy for the client, the nurse will plan each experience so that Miss J will not become fatigued or saturated with learning activities. As Miss J progresses, her accomplishments will change so that when she is visited at home it can be expected that by the second week Miss J will be able to prepare her own meals according to her prescribed diabetic diet.

All of the above expected outcomes have time limitations or "givens" that clearly define *when* the terminal behavior will occur. All are intended to evaluate Miss J's progress in learning diabetic care. They also are intended to measure the effectiveness of the nurse's attempts to teach Miss J. Learning diabetic care is the long-term expectation; whereas the four stated expectations are the short-term means of measuring the long-term goal.

The third factor that Mager deems essential for describing terminal behavior is the criterion for acceptable performance. Probably the most obvious way to indicate an acceptable performance is to specify the lower limits of the performance. Time limits, minimum number of correct responses, important characteristics, and accuracy are measures of acceptable performance. For example, Mr. K will demonstrate comfort during sleep when he can decrease his number of coughing episodes to no more than four between the hours of twelve and four in the morning. The acceptable performance for Mr. K is when he can demonstrate comfortable sleep, which is defined as his ability to decrease his coughing episodes to less than four. The restrictions on his performance are the hours between twelve and four when he must decrease his coughing. The criterion of acceptable performance describes how well the expected behavior will be performed.

Sometimes an expected outcome is so stated that it is difficult to decide whether a phrase is a restriction or a criterion for acceptable performance. If the phrase says anything about the excellence of the performance, it is a criterion. If it is difficult to distinguish, no harm is done so long as the outcome is clearly communicated. After all, the important matter is not the label but how well the evaluation criterion performs the function for which it is intended.

Although each of the items discussed makes an expected outcome more specific, it is not necessary to include all items in each evaluative criterion. The intent is to write terminal criteria that communicate the expected outcome of the nursing action so that all those involved in the client's care will be able to determine if the care has accomplished what it was designed to do.

A final consideration in writing terminal expectations is that the nurse should remember to define the statement in terms of the client's cultural and social patterns. It is difficult to achieve some goals when the very goal is in opposition to the client's cultural response. In some ethnic groups, moaning and thrashing about when in pain are expected. If the nurse expects this person to demonstrate comfort by a decrease in noise making and a lessening of facial and body movements, the expectation will not be met. But this does not necessarily mean the pain is not decreased. Terminal behaviors are defined in terms that fit the client's individual cultural framework.

It is time for nurses to recognize the importance and necessity of structuring and formulating evaluation criteria in client-centered behavioral terms. Nurses can discard the attitude that professional tasks possess ethereal qualities or that there are some intangible aspects in nursing care that just cannot be evaluated. Performance in nursing can be observed and evaluated if the nurse identifies the expected behavior and describes the conditions or the criteria of acceptance under which the performance will occur.

The process of planning nursing care is never ending. The dynamic nature of man and his ever-changing world demands continuous planning so that nursing care equilibrates the client's needs. The following examples illustrate the process in totality.

Example 1.

Assessment: Tommy, a 2-year-old child with measles who convulses with high temperatures, has a temperature of 104° F.

Stress: Viral agent (measles).

Response: Rise in temperature, the result of antimicrobial action of the body; possible convulsions with high temperatures.

Problem: How to reduce Tommy's temperature before he convulses?

Priority order of selected nursing actions:
1. Give Tommy two grains of aspirin rectally.
2. Submerge Tommy's entire body in tepid water.
3. Maintain a cool but draft-free environment.

Evaluation criteria:
1. Within 20 minutes of sponging, Tommy's temperature will be at least two degrees lower than it was when sponging began (104° F).
2. Within one hour Tommy's temperature will measure between 100° and 101° F rectally.

Example 2.

Assessment: Mrs. K, who is 67-years-old, is 2 days postsurgical for abdominal adhesions. She is developing pulmonary congestion but refuses to cough because her abdominal area hurts when she coughs.

Stress: Surgery.

Response: Abdominal pain; pulmonary congestion.

Problem: How to get Mrs. K to produce a productive cough without experiencing severe abdominal pain?

Priority order of selected nursing actions:

1. Find out if Mrs. K knows why she is asked to cough.
2. If necessary, explain the need to cough postsurgically.
3. Splint Mrs. K's abdomen with a pillow and have her cough deeply. Repeat until she produces sputum.

Evaluation criterion:

After the nurse splints her abdomen, Mrs. K will cough deeply without pain until she is able to bring up sputum.

Although the process of planning nursing care presented in this book takes time and energy, there is no substitute for its value to the practitioner in developing quality nursing care.[10] Every nurse can acquire the ability to create innovative approaches to client and community problems once she begins to deliberately and critically analyze actions before implementation, rather than after. The satisfaction and sense of accomplishment realized from a nursing plan that helps the client reach high-level wellness in an individualized manner is well worth the extra time and energy expended.

SUMMARY

During the third phase of nursing care planning, the nurse formulates a plan for action. Alternative approaches and their consequences are considered. The probability of occurrence of each consequence is estimated, as are the value and risk. After analyzing each consequence's probability of occurrence, value, and risk, using the guidelines for decision making, a nursing approach is selected. Having selected an approach, it is then necessary for the nurse to devise a plan for evaluation. This plan is the fourth and final phase of the planning of nursing care and is composed of a description of the terminal expectations. The evaluation plan includes a description of:

1. The specific behavior that will be accepted as evidence of the desired outcome
2. The important conditions under which the behavior will occur
3. The criterion of acceptable performance

Priority setting of nursing actions is essential if lives are to be saved and delivery of quality care is to be assured. Goals, timing, maximum therapeutic effects, and policies determine the priority of actions.

The key to quality nursing care lies in the nurse's desire, interest, and

---

[10]The decision-making process presented here has been developed by the San Jose State College Nursing faculty. It is part of a curriculum revision funded by United States Public Health grant 5-D10-NU-00292-04.

ability to systematically plan care. A process that includes comprehensive assessment, accurate problem identification, plans for action, and an evaluation based on the desired outcome is the most efficient and practical way to plan nursing care.

Planned nursing care culminates in a nursing care plan. Chapter Five explores the content, practicality, and use of a care plan and will point out its major value as a means of providing continuity in nursing care.

Suggested readings

Banathy, Bela H.: Instructional systems, Belmont, 1968, Fearon Publishers, p. 33.

Bloom, B. S., and Krathwohl, P. R.: Taxonomy of educational objectives handbook I, cognitive domain, New York, 1956, David McKay Co., Inc.

Clissold, Grace K., and Metz, Edith A.: Evaluation—a tangible process, Nurs. Outlook **14**(3):41-45, 1966.

Gagné, Robert W.: The condition of learning, New York, 1965, Holt, Rinehart & Winston, Inc., pp. 156-170.

Gagné, Robert W.: Educational objectives and human performance. In Krumboltz, J. D., editor: Learning and the educational process, Chicago, 1965, Rand McNally & Co., p. 12.

Geitgey, Doris A., and Crowley, Dorothy: Preparing objectives, Amer. J. Nurs. **65**(1):95-97, 1965.

Hall, Jay, O'Leary, Vincent, and Williams, Martha: The decision-making grid: a model of decision-making styles, California Management Review **7**(2):43-54, 1964.

Kerlinger, Fred: Foundation of behavioral research, New York, 1965, Holt, Rinehart & Winston, Inc., pp. 117-119.

Mager, Robert: Preparing instructional objectives, Belmont, 1962, Fearon Publishers.

McDonald, Frederick J., and Harms, Mary T.: Theoretical model for an experimental curriculum, Nurs. Outlook **14**(8):48-51, 1966.

Smith, Dorothy: Writing objectives as a nursing practice skill, Amer. J. Nurs. **71**(2):319-320, 1971.

Tyler, Ralph W.: Some persistent questions on the defining of objectives. In Lindvall, C. M., editor: Defining educational objectives, Pittsburgh, 1964, University of Pittsburgh Press.

Chapter

5

A MEANS OF IMPLEMENTING THE PLANNED CARE:
A NURSING CARE PLAN

What you plan for one step may affect what will be done at another
one . . . during your planning, other ideas, facts or examples may
come to mind. . . . Be sure to write them down.

Jerrold Kemp[1]

OVERVIEW

All those who administer, supervise, and teach nursing care agree that
planning care is an essential part of the practice of nursing. Care plans that
record and communicate the planned care are equally important. They are
the *tools* for providing coordination and continuity of care. Care plans are an
excellent means of keeping the care individualized and current. Like the
familiar "medicine card" the care plan also offers safety to the client; it is a
practical and accessible place for making notations about precautions, specific
limitations, and suggested approaches for each client. The purpose of this
chapter is twofold:

1. To present the nursing care plan as a tool for providing individualized,
   comprehensive, safe, and coordinated care
2. To explore various ways of developing and revising the care plan

EVOLUTION OF NURSING CARE PLANS

After the second world war with the onset of the team approach to
nursing care came the need for better communication and a unified plan of
action. Since several persons were involved in the care of one person, some
means of communicating the nursing needs and nursing interventions to all
members of the nursing team was needed. The written care plan was devised

---

[1] Kemp, Jerrold: Instructional design, Belmont, 1971, Fearon Publishers, p. 11.

as a method for communicating the nursing care activities of each client to all members of the nursing team. It was also viewed as a tool for evaluating nursing approaches. *Patient-centered care* became the byword as more and more was said about the need for care that was individualized, consistent, and provided continuity. Updating care plans to meet the changing needs of the client became the impetus to the team conference.

By the late 1950's nursing care plans were still being utilized mostly as a tool for improving communication within the nursing team; but after 1960 another dimension appeared. Nurses began to place emphasis on assessment. According to Bernice Wagner, the nursing care plan was "a portrait—a picture of him [the client] as a person, of the kind of care he needs, of the goals which nursing personnel hope to attain for him."[2] Objectives for care were included and suggested ways of moving the client toward these goals were outlined as well as a means for evaluating goal attainment. Although the nursing care plan was a well-accepted concept within the nursing profession, there were some indications that nurses were having difficulty utilizing the tool. Most nursing care plans consisted of notations of medical orders, whereas the client's emotional, spiritual, and psychological needs were almost ignored.[3] Long- and short-term goals were absent or unrealistic.[4]

During the late 1960's and early 1970's efforts have been made to expand the use of nursing care plans. A circular nursing care plan was proposed and tried. The plan was initiated by the nurse in the intake clinic where the client was first seen. It then accompanied the client into the hospital and out again into the community. In this instance the nursing care plan not only served as a communicative tool, but also provided health personnel with the client's history and health plan for use in continuing care.[5] There were now three dimensions in planning supplied by the care plan: communication, individualization, and continuity. However, additional dimensions of care, which greatly increase efficiency, are part of the nursing care plan.

PURPOSES OF NURSING CARE PLAN

Nursing care planning, when carried to completion, culminates in the written nursing care plan. The plan includes the client's needs and problems, the priorities that have been set, the approaches that have been selected, and the evaluative criteria to measure the actions. As Nancy Kelly states:

---

[2]Wagner, Bernice: Care plans—right, reasonable and reachable, Amer. J. Nurs. 69(5):986, 1969.

[3]Kelly, Nancy: Nursing care plans, Nurs. Outlook 14(5):61, 1966.

[4]Grosichi, J. P., and others: Nursing care plans—survey of status and opinions about current usage, J. Psychiat. Nurs. 5(6):567-585, 1967.

[5]Sweet, P. R., and Stark, Irmagene: The circular nursing care plan, Amer. J. Nurs. 70(6):1300. 1970.

A well-written plan provides a central source of information about the patient and a description of his nursing needs. . . . A nursing care plan does not insure optimal patient care, but it will never be attained without a plan.[6]

The nursing care plan is a personalized account that indicates the kind of nursing needed for the particular client. It reflects the objectives or goals of the nursing care and is not merely a list of nursing activities. As outlined by Thora Kron, the aim or objective of the nursing care plan is based on three components:

1. Medical care prescribed by the physician
2. General care, which may be determined by the client's health problem or by the agency's policy
3. Nursing care that the nurse, functioning as an independent practitioner, determines is necessary to help the client cope with his health problem or his treatment[7]

Nursing care plans have many purposes. They provide for:

1. Individualized care
2. Continuity of care
3. Communication of care
4. Evaluation of care
5. Comprehensive care
6. Coordination of care
7. Team spirit

Individualized care

Nursing care plans that include the client's needs, problems, priorities, and selected approaches demonstrate individualized care. It is true that many nursing activities are uniform in that they are used with many clients. The uniqueness of these generalized nurse behaviors is that they are selected for a particular individual to solve a particular problem, since the concept of individual care is based on the belief that each person is unique in some special way. Each individual, although he may experience the same assault from a virus or a social stress as another, responds to his total experience in a separate and individual manner. Values, expectations, and differing life experiences create and reinforce these differences in man.

An expanding awareness by nurses of the need for individualized care has made planning an essential and central part of nursing practice. It has encouraged nurses to consider the dimensions of prevention and rehabilitation as well as cure. It has emphasized the need for client involvement. For

---

[6] Kelly: Nursing care plans, p. 61.

[7] Kron, Thora: Nursing team leadership, Philadelphia, 1961, W. B. Saunders Company, pp. 133-134.

who knows more about the client than himself? The concept of individualized care has also placed major emphasis on the rights and privileges of each person. Not only does the client have the right to seek care but he also has the right to expect a reasonably comfortable and dignified death. He has the right to refuse care or to demand certain types of care as long as it fits into his therapeutic regimen. It also means the client's past, present, and future are considered as the plan is developed. Why plan an approach when knowledge that it will not work is available from the client?

How, then, does the nurse plan individualized care for a client in an agency that has rigid limitations? How can nurses find time to individualize care? Individualized care does not mean laissez-faire scheduling or chaos. On the contrary, it demands regular and systematic planning—planning within the schedule of the institution. More than anything, individualized care means that the care is designed to meet the needs of the client and is delivered within the restrictions or limitations of the institution. For instance, most hospitals have fairly rigid schedules. These are necessary or there would be no way for the many people who need care to receive it. But even within these tight limitations the nurse has the flexibility to plan bathing procedures, activities, treatments, meals, and visiting hours to fit the individualized schedule of the client. Most of the current trends toward a loosening of hospital rigidity are because of nurses who have become involved in helping to provide more flexibility for individualized care. Individualizing care does take a bit longer than routine administration of care, but with team involvement and practice the process becomes exciting and very rewarding. Many nurses can attest to the fact that in the long run the little time spent in individualizing care saves much time that would have been spent in coping with clients who demand attention and complain about a lack of individualized care.

Continuity of care

The written nursing care plan provides for continuity; it provides for an even flow or progression of care from one nurse to another, from one shift to another, from one discipline to another. When more then one person is involved in the delivery of care, a written care plan is absolutely essential if duplication, omissions, and errors are to be avoided. Care plans that provide for continuity of care include: (1) long-term and short-term goals; (2) information about the client's desires, preferences, and expectations; (3) information about the client's problems, the proposed approaches, and the *pattern* of care.

Care plans that identify the task to be accomplished and how the task might be carried out are of particular benefit to personnel unfamiliar with the client. New personnel, float staff, or persons with varying degrees of preparation find their task not only easier but also much more satisfying when goals and notations of progress are part of the care plan. When the speech therapist or the occupational therapist has clearly outlined the ultimate goals and the expected rate of progress, as well as limitations that might influence the progress, the nursing staff can supplement the therapy by participating constructively in the client's plan of care. In order for continuity of care to occur, systematic communication must be practiced.

Without continuity of care there is the possibility that gaps may occur. Suppose Mr. Green is 2 days postoperative and has an order for progressive activity. Unless there is some notation of what Mr. Green has accomplished the day before, the nurse might assume he dangled his feet over the edge of the bed the first day and he will sit up today. On the other hand, if the goal of progressive activity has been determined and a schedule proposed, it becomes a simple task to carry out the nursing actions in sequence. The same is true if the nurse presumes the client had preoperative teaching about the postoperative period. A care plan that outlines the preoperative teaching gives the nurse a clear idea of what to expect postoperatively.

Communication of care

One of the most important and vital purposes of the nursing care plan is its use as a communicative tool. The written plan provides data about the client's condition and previous care and becomes a resource to refer to at any time during his care. It is an excellent way of conveying accurate information about the status of the client, and is therefore one way of alleviating hearsay and distortions in communication. The written care plan provides information to many persons: the nurse, the physician, ancillary team members, the client and his family, and all other personnel involved in the client's care (such as laboratory technicians, x-ray technicians, dietary workers, social workers, and others). Regardless of the setting the nursing care plan should be available to all those involved in the care.

The nurse who is directly responsible for the care is particularly interested in the care plan. Although the nurse may not have instituted the plan, a glance at it orients her to the situation, or it may bring her up to date if there has been a time lag since the last contact. Without a written account, the nurse would need to rely on memory or on the verbal descriptions of others. Such verbal accounts become more and more distorted as the number of persons involved increases. When more than one nurse shares the client's care, the written care plan acts as a relay system. It records changes in the client's condition, his current responses, the kinds of nursing approaches used, and the goals for therapy.

Quite often the nursing care plan is supplemented by a verbal interpretation as the nurse transfers the responsibility of care to another. But for maximum benefit to both the client and those involved in his care, a nursing care plan should communicate the client's status and the nursing care needed without added explanation. One very useful means of updating the nursing care plan in a busy hospital, so that it becomes a functional tool for the delivery of nursing care, is to do "nursing rounds." By visiting each client with the care plan the nurse is able to validate the plan or make changes as needed. The client becomes an integral part of the plan as he discusses his condition with the nurse. Observations are made, questions are answered, and the client's complaints and concerns are given attention. Problems are verified, goals are clarified, and a general evaluation of progress is made. All pertinent and helpful information is noted on the care plan and changes are made at the bedside. No time lapses between the time the client makes a statement and the nurse can return to the nursing station, therefore there is less chance for confusion about what the client requested or shared with the nurse. And since the total nursing team is present, there is less chance for mixed messages from the nurse to the team members.

There is nothing as reassuring as a nurse who takes the time with the rest of the nursing team to visit each client to update the nursing care plans. It tells the client that he is a distinct person, that the team does care what he thinks and feels, that he is part of the planned care, and that the nurse is assuming responsibility for quality care. A similar type of updating or means of keeping the care plan current and moving in the proper direction is the case summary. Many community health nurses, clinic nurses, and industrial nurses utilize the summary method. At the end of each visit the nurse outlines the visit by writing down (1) the purpose of the visit, (2) the goals of care, (3) the observations and information gained from the visit, (4) the progress (goal attainment) since the last visit, (5) any new needs or problems, and (6) goals for the next visit. Here again a critique of the client's progress is made in light of his needs and his progress toward need gratification. With this kind of summary the client could be transferred to any other health worker, who would have a clear picture of what had occurred so far and what goals for therapy were recommended. Persons called upon for consultation find such a summary very helpful.

Just as the client is part of the care plan, so is the client's family. Families are an important factor in the client's response to a health problem and in his ability to cope. Families are also an excellent source of information. Too often they are excluded from the scene at a time when their presence may be needed. If they are to be supportive and actively involved in the care, they need to be apprised of the direction of the therapy. Even if they opt not to be actively involved they have the right to know what is being done and why. When family members do become involved in the care they must know how they can most appropriately participate. It is an old story to see a devoted and loving mother undo all the progress toward independence that the nursing staff has so painstakingly developed, without knowing she is violating the goals of treatment. Without knowledge of the goals and the therapeutic plan, the family member may be unwittingly working at cross purposes with the nursing staff. When the nursing goals are shared, the family not only *feels* it is part of the care but it is also better prepared to contribute in an appropriate and helpful manner.

A major reason for involving the family in the care is that many of the client's health problems will need to be handled at home. Hospitalization time is becoming shorter, with generative, supportive, and protective care occurring at home. Therefore, it is imperative that the family not only be kept abreast of the therapeutic plan, but also actively participate in the planning and implementation of the care. Many factors influence the degree of involvement members of a family are able (or even want) to accept. Whenever a member shows interest the nurse should reinforce his attempts and encourage his participation. Some members want to help but are reluctant to get involved because they fear they are interfering. Nurses can listen and watch for cues that indicate interest. Sensitivity to others and their needs is a vital and extremely useful skill that nurses use when assessing clients. The same skill is useful as nurses relate with families.

Nursing care plans can be an important adjunct to the physician. They serve to give him information of the client's needs, adding to the data he already has. This accumulation of data enables him to individualize the medical therapy. There are times when the nurse needs the medical expertise of the physician and it is at these times that the written care plan acts as a reminder; questions can be answered, perceptions validated, and approaches clarified as the nurse and the physician discuss the plan of care. Such a collaborative approach to health care results in a more efficient and economical utilization of the physician's and the nurse's knowledge and skills, while providing maximum care for the client.

Clients are frequently transferred from one unit to another, one agency to another, one health worker to another. Concomitant to their mobility in care is the increasing number of persons involved at any one time in their care. With so much mobility and exposure to so many personnel, it seems obvious that a written plan of care is needed. Easy exchange of information is possible when a care plan is kept up to date. Duplication, omissions, and discrepancies can be avoided if the person assuming responsibility for care knows about the client's problems (solved and unsolved), his strengths, responses, and those nursing interventions that seemed successful. All of this can be conveyed in a care plan. It is unfair to expect the new health worker to individualize care with little or no data with which to work. It is equally unfair to expect the client to adjust to a whole new approach of care. With any change, whether it be an adjustment to new personnel or to a new setting, there is energy diverted from the process of healing and recovery to coping with the change. In some instances, the client cannot afford the dissipation of such energy. But if the client can see that his needs, his problems, and his progress are being communicated to the new personnel, some of his tension may be reduced. Time is saved, anxiety reduced, and efficiency increased when a current and complete nursing care plan accompanies the transferred client.

Whenever possible, a verbal dialogue between the two persons providing the care is warranted, since such interchange strengthens the communicative bonds between health workers and helps insure continuity of care.

Nursing care plans can become part of the nursing history. Like the client's chart, his hospital records, and his medical history, the care plan can be useful in planning care with successive health problems. The previous nursing care plan may indicate some of the client's responses, problems encountered, and approaches that did and did not work. Great caution must be exercised, though, that the previous plan is not taken at face value. Old records should be used as supplementary data, that is, as information from which to build a *new* plan of care. People change, medical and surgical care improves, knowledge expands, and so should the plan for nursing care. The well-written, up-to-date, and complete nursing care plan goes a long way toward helping the nurse who assumes responsibility for care to proceed in an orderly and productive fashion, even though the data received will eventually be validated. It is always better to begin with something than to blunder along with nothing.

Evaluation of care

Nursing care plans provide a vehicle for evaluating nursing care. If the nurse or other members of the health team consistently keep the plan current it provides a means of evaluating the care. Evaluation is an ongoing process that occurs each time someone writes down a goal, an approach, and a response to that approach. Certain nursing actions will help the client become more comfortable, more at ease, more informed. Others will not. Unless nursing actions are evaluated, no one will know which actions produced desired effects. Evaluation of the efficiency of present nursing actions is the realistic appraisal for making deliberate change. In evaluating the care of a client the nurse seeks evidence that the problem has been solved and data to determine if there are any new needs or problems. To accomplish this twofold evaluative process the goals, actions, and evaluative criteria are included in the plan of care. Continuous evaluation keeps the care plan functional. There is nothing as frustrating as a care plan that states that the client desires his sleeping pill at 10 PM before retiring and then discovering that the client is no longer taking any medication for sleep.

When several persons are caring for one client, knowledge of whether certain nursing measures have been effective or ineffective is liable to get lost unless the information is recorded in the care plan. By providing information on goals, actions, and responses in the nursing care plan, the client can benefit from the evaluative actions of many. From this material commonalities and recurring patterns of response emerge, which permit the nurse to be consistent and definitive in the delivery of care.

Comprehensive care

Nursing care plans that provide comprehensiveness include care for the whole person. Man's psychic, social, physical, and emotional needs are considered. His total response to stress, his cultural and ethnic reactions, and his biochemical processes are assessed, if the care plan is to be anything more than a list of the physician's orders. Too often a review of existing care plans reveals a sad and degenerating trend.

> For twenty years the nursing care planning concept has been accepted in principle. However, despite considerable impetus nursing care plans are incomplete or non-existent in a majority of patient care settings in this study . . . with minor exceptions [they] did not reflect a comprehensive approach to patient care.[8]

Care planning that utilizes the stress-response model presented in Chapter Three enables the nurse to define problems and decide on actions that are holistic. Care that only focuses on the client's disease process or on the physician's orders is only partial care. It is like anticipating a full eight-course dinner and receiving only the soup and salad. You go away hungry and feel only partially satisfied and very cheated. Nursing care that does not provide comprehensiveness does not give the client what he desires, what he needs, or what he should receive.

Comprehensive care is often best accomplished when the health team gets together to plan care. Team conferences for planning care can include only the nursing staff or, to be more inclusive, have a multidisciplinary makeup. Since the activities involved in developing the nursing care plan tend to affect all those who carry out direct care (nonprofessionals) as well as those who direct the care (that is, registered nurses), all should be present. Each has something to offer, whether it is an observation, a first-hand account, or data from the family. As they pool data to identify problems or to modify approaches, there develops a sense of satisfaction as contributions are accepted and ideas incorporated. Skill in observation and communication improves as the team members are caught up in the process of gathering data. By listening and conferring with one another to build the plan of care, each begins to see how the pieces fit—how the observations of one member coupled with the scientific knowledge of another provide a clearer more comprehensive picture.

---

[8]Cuica, Rudolph: An analysis of nursing care plans in selected bay area community hospitals. Unpublished master's thesis, San Jose State College, June 1971, p. 67.

Coordination of care

The concept of coordination, like continuity, is concerned with the even flow of health care. When nurses coordinate nursing care they arrange the therapeutic plan so that the client's energy, comfort, and dignity are preserved. Timing and synchronizing schedules, conveying information, and proper preparation effect the manner in which the client's care plan is arranged. Nurses often schedule treatments or synchronize nursing care with visits or arrange the client's time so that maximum benefit can be gained from the therapy without undue inconvenience. Some diagnostic tests require fasting and therefore should be scheduled early in the morning. Some treatments create fatigue and should be scheduled when the client is well rested. Others are scheduled on certain days because of departmental limitations. The same is true of various types of therapy. Factors such as pain, boredom, fatigue, and expense are considered when coordinating care. Is it better to schedule all the tests to be done at one time and shorten the time required, or is it better to spread out the tests and conserve the client's energy? Is it better to schedule the diagnostic x-rays for the morning when the client is fresh and alert, or to wait until the afternoon after he has rested in the morning? And what about the various departments? What are they to do if every nurse decides to schedule in the morning? These questions and many others arise when decisions need to be made about coordinating care. Nurses need to know the policies of other departments and the preferences of other health workers when coordinating care if the care is to proceed smoothly. Much of the coordination of care depends on communicating the plan to nonnursing services and to other professionals. The nursing care plan is a convenient means for communicating the total plan of care. Just as the care plan is available to other departments and nonnursing professionals for information, it is also an excellent place for their comments and progress reports. Such contributions add to the comprehensiveness of the plan and at the same time give data for improving coordination of care.

Coordination of care is particularly needed when more than one service or one professional is responsible for the same area of care. Suppose the physician, the nurse, the anesthesiologist, and the physiotherapist are involved in teaching the client about postoperative exercises. Unless a unified approach in both content and technique is used, the client is liable to become confused. When all involved are aware of the goals and of the successful approaches, time is saved, the client is provided with consistency, and the goals are more likely to be met. Nursing care plans can provide this unified approach. It must be remembered, though, if more than one person or department is involved in the same aspect of care that responsibility, as well as sequence, must be established. Interdisciplinary conferences in which each person can contribute his ideas and knowledge help considerably when planning teaching approaches and determining responsibility.

Team spirit

Another reason for making a nursing care plan is that it promotes team work. As each person involved in the client's care contributes to the care plan he finds himself to be a part of a larger whole. Working together the health team shares its ideas, observations, and suggestions about the client and participates in selecting nursing approaches. This participation in the plan of care creates a sense of responsibility in the team members for the delivery of care because they shared in the process of planning that care; it also promotes a sense of team spirit for the same reason. As the team continues to work together to plan care, it begins to see the benefit of a team effort. The client becomes the recipient of the cooperative effort of several persons. But teamwork is not enough unless the product of team effort is somehow made accessible to all concerned. The planning is either recorded in writing, taped on a recorder, or stored in a computer for retrieval. Somehow the plan of care must be available so that continuous care can be provided.

The nursing care plan is a guide to the care *currently* being given the client and cannot therefore take the place of the client's chart, which is a record of the care that has been given. If the care plan is to stimulate unity and provide quality nursing care, it must be complete, current, and available for all to use.

ELEMENTS OF THE CARE PLAN

Many formats for nursing care plans are used for implementing the planned nursing care. Some have sections for the physician's orders, the treatments, and medication, leaving other space for the nursing objectives and approaches. Regardless of the format there are certain essential elements that must be included in the plan if individualized and comprehensive care is to be given. These include:

1. Personal data about the client
2. The schedule of the client's basic daily care, which includes his treatments, medications, and appointments for diagnostic tests, treatments in other departments, or consultation with other professionals
3. The identified needs and problems of the client, with both long-term and short-term goals
4. The planned approaches for care
5. The evaluative criteria of this planned care

The format can be as innovative and creative as needed, but should include the above elements and provide ample space for each.

Personal data

Certain information about the client is needed on every nursing care plan. His name, age, marital status, identifying number, occupation, admitting diagnosis, religion, and his surgical procedure and its date (if any) should be stated. Data about his family, such as closest relative, are not always necessary but if the nursing history indicates that this information is important as part of the client's personal data, it should be included. Specialized areas, such as the obstetrical unit, will want additional information. Data about the client's number of pregnancies (gravida), her number of living children (para), and whether she will breast or bottle feed her baby are all a part of the needed personal data. Although this information is not directly a part of the plan, it is important because it provides background material that will help the nurse understand the client better and therefore help create an individualized plan of care.

Schedule of basic daily care

If the care plan is to be functional it should include a description of the client's daily care. Information about diet, activity, medications,[9] treatments, and personal hygiene are transcribed from the physician's orders to the plan of care. The client's sleeping habits, fluid preferences, elimination patterns, dietary practices, and degree of self-care that are obtained during the nursing history are also included. If the client is scheduled for therapy in some other department or is receiving services from other professionals, these data are noted, including when and where the event will occur.

Some logical or sequential ordering of these data is necessary if the plan of care is to provide a complete picture of the total care of the client. The greatest advances toward organizing a plan of care have been with computerized nursing care plans.[10] Each day's activity schedule is printed out the night before. Information on the client's activity limitations, treatments, diagnostic tests, meals, and other specialized therapies are entered into the computer and are returned in a summarized hourly itemized schedule of events. Since computers are very expensive and not available to many hospitals or convalescent units, a similar type of care plan can be developed and be included in the familiar Kardex. Fig. 10 is an example of a written plan of care, with all events itemized and inserted in their proper time slot. If this type of care plan is to be used it is essential that it be renewed at the close of each nursing shift. Adjustments, additions, and deletions are necessary if the care plan is to remain current and usable.

Identified needs and problems (current and potential)

A nursing care plan that includes stated needs and problems provides the nurse with valuable information for the development of individualized

---

[9]Since most hospitals use medicine cards for each medication, there is no need to enter the specific medication and its route of administration on the care plan. The time for administration is all that is recorded on the care plan.

[10]Cornell, Sadie H., and Brush, Frances: Systems approach to nursing care plans, Amer. J. Nurs. **71**(7):1376-1378, 1971.

DATE: *Jan. 18, 1972*					
NAME: *Edith Johnson*		HYGIENE: *Bed Bath*	TREATMENTS:		LAB TESTS & X-RAY:
AGE: *68*		ACTIVITY: *Bedrest*	I.P.P.B.		*CBC, Lytes in A.M.*
		DIET: *Liquid*	T, C & D.B.		*Chest X-ray*
DIAGNOSIS:			I.V. #4, 1000 cc		
Cholelithiasis			D5-W c̄ 0.45 NaCl		

SURGERY: *Jan 17, 1972*	TIME	LOCATION	ACTIVITY	BY WHOM	COMMENTS
Cholecystectomy	7:00 A.M.	*Nursing Unit*	*Lab-work*	*lab technician*	*N.P.O.*
DATE OF DELIVERY:	7:30		*V.S.*	*nurse aide*	
	8:00	*Nursing Unit*	*Breakfast*		*likes apple juice for break-fast, needs help.*
PARA:	8:30				
	9:00	*Nursing Unit X-ray Dept.*	*medication X-ray client*	*R.N. X-ray tech.*	*Provide client with pajama pants.*
GRAVIDA:	9:30				
RELIGION:	10:00	*Nursing Unit*	*Bed-bath*	*nurse aide*	*have client T, C & D.B. Prefers to lie flat – no pillows*
Catholic	10:30	*Nursing Unit*	*I.P.P.B.*	*inhalation therapist*	*client becomes frightened and needs to rest p̄ 5 min.*
DATE OF ADMISSION:	11:00				
Jan. 14, 1972	11:30	*Nursing Unit*	*V.S.*	*nurse aide*	
	12:00	*Nursing Unit*	*Lunch*		*needs help*
SHIFT: *7-3*	12:30				
	1:00	*Nursing Unit*	*Medication*	*R.N.*	*likes grape juice in styrofoam*
	1:30	*Nursing Unit*	*I.V. complete superimpose #5*	*R.N.*	
	2:00				
	2:30	*Nursing Unit*	*I.P.P.B.*	*inhalation therapist*	*rest p̄ 5 min. to reduce fear – stay to her until she is calm & breathing regularly.*
	3:00				

Fig. 10. Scheduled-event card.

nursing approaches. Clearly stated needs enable the nurse to select activities to meet a specific purpose. The same is true of nursing problems. When they are written in specific terms the nurse is able to design a nursing strategy to promote change or to support the client's current coping behavior. Nursing care plans that state needs and problems let everyone involved in the care know how the individual is coping with his present stress situation. Interviews with the client's family and friends and a review of his chart, as well as communication with the individual, give the nurse data about how he views his situation; such data as what factors precipitated the situation and what he expects as a result need to be clarified. The client's expectations are important because they help the nurse to know what to reinforce and what to change. When the expectations are realistic, the nurse can plan approaches to meet them; when they are unrealistic a problem exists and the nurse will plan care accordingly.

Potential as well as current needs and problems are included in the care plan. For example, a baby with hyaline membrane disease has a current need for respiratory assistance. Actions will be selected to promote adequate O_2-CO_2 exchange and to help him cope with the potential drying effect of inhalation therapy provided by intermittent possitive pressure devices. Another client is hospitalized because of extreme anxiety. He paces endlessly, talks incessantly, and cannot sleep. The nurse who plans his care should institute actions to handle his need for rest, as well as his potential need for adequate nutrition and elimination. Notations of current and potential needs such as these help the nurse plan observations and actions to assist the client in coping with his health problems as they change. When potential problems are considered, prevention becomes the focus, with many actions designed to handle current problems so that future problems will not arise. A great advantage to considering potential problems is that the nurse is ready for what might occur.

Planned approaches for care

After decisions have been made about nursing approaches they are listed opposite the nursing needs and problems. The nurse who is responsible for maintaining the care plan writes and updates the nursing problems and approaches. The selected approaches, which are directives, communicate to all personnel what the plan of care is intended to do and the means for accomplishing the intent. But if these actions are not clearly stated they will have minimal effect. For instance, such statements as "offer emotional support" and "force fluids" do not specifically tell the nurse what to do. Misunderstandings, misinterpretations, and confusion occur if the statement of action is not clearly and descriptively written. When a satisfactory approach is determined through discussion during the team conference, it is written so there is no possible way to misunderstand the prescribed action. The statement of the nursing action describes: (1) what will be done, (2) how the action will be carried out, and (3) when the action will occur. When the nursing action statement clearly indicates *what* the nurse is to do, it indicates a satisfactory approach has been found. This does not negate the possibility that another approach may be tried but means that a particular action is available and has demonstrated some success. Instead of writing "offer support" the nursing action could read, "listen to Mrs. Green's proposed plans and reinforce any decisions she makes about returning home." In this particular example the "support" offered is directed toward what the person (Mrs. Green) needs and desires; support in this case is helping Mrs. Green make a decision. If and when it seems necessary to support a client, the statement indicates clearly what is to be supported and how it can be done.

Some actions require observational skills. Ongoing assessment and evaluation depend on observational nursing actions. Unless the action is described so that the essential factors pertaining to the client's condition are noted, the observer will not know what to look for. Some direction for what the observer is to do if the observation demonstrates a significant change will also be included in the statement. For example, if the nursing action states "check the apical heart beat every hour and report to the physician any reading over 180/min. or under 80/min.," the nurse knows exactly what to look for, what is acceptable performance, what is a deviation, and what to report. If, however, the observation reveals no problems, reporting what was discovered belongs in the client's chart and with the team leader. Occasionally a nursing action directs the nurse to look for the presence or absence of some sign or symptom. A nursing statement that says "check the pulse for irregularity and report the presence or absence to the team leader" clearly tells the nurse what specifically should be done.

Statements of nursing actions that describe *how* the nurse will act are one way of providing continuity and individuality in care. The nurse knows by reading the nursing action statement exactly what is expected and what the client needs or desires. It is unfair to expect the client to tell every person who cares for him that he likes things a certain way. For instance, if the client in the hospital wants a small light on every night and his pillows arranged in a certain way, this information is included in the nursing action statement. Or if a client in the home likes his dressings done at a certain time and in a particular way, the nursing action indicates when and how the client prefers the procedure to be accomplished. To assume that these particular desires will be passed on by word of mouth is invalid.

An important element of the how in a nursing statement is the amount of assistance the client needs. How much help does the nurse give the client? Can he help at all or is he totally reliant on the nurse to meet his needs? If he can help, what can he do? If he can do most of the care, what care does the nurse need to provide? An example of each of these statements that describe total, partial, and no help might be:

> **Total care:** Give a full bed bath, the client is unable to help.
>
> **Partial care:** Give the bed bath, letting the client wash his arms, chest, face, and genitalia. You will need to do his back, legs, and feet. Set him in a chair while you make the bed.
>
> **No help:** Give the client his bath supplies. He can bathe himself. Make his bed as he ambulates about the room.

The *when* of a nursing statement indicates the frequency and time of the action. Statements that specify the time of the action eliminate omissions and gaps in care. If the nursing action reads "sitz bath B.I.D.," there is the chance that it will not be done at all or that it will be done more than twice a day, since there is no way of knowing from this statement when the sitz bath was or is to be given. "Give a sitz bath after the morning bath and before bed at night" indicates exactly when the nursing action is to be carried out. If the nursing action statement says "once daily," it is very possible that it may be forgotten entirely, if each nursing shift believes the other is responsible. Assigning a particular time to a nursing action alleviates the problem of

DATE: 1/18/72		
NAME: Mrs. Edith Johnson	DIAGNOSIS: Cholelithiasis	
DOCTOR: Dr. Gordon Knowles	SURGERY: Cholecystectomy	DATE OF SURGERY: 1/17/72

CLIENT NEEDS/PROBLEMS In Priority Order	NURSING APPROACH	EXPECTED OUTCOME
1. Having a lot of pain - doesn't ask for pain med.	1. Give pain medication by hypo every three hours from last injection (don't wait until she asks)	1. ½ hour p̄ medication, she looks more comfortable and states she feels free of pain and remains that way for at least 3 hours
2. She is worried about her husband who lives alone and needs help with meals.	2. Talk to V.N.A. coordinator this A.M. to arrange help for Mr. Johnson.	2. The V.N.A. nurse will arrange for a home health aide to visit Mr. Johnson daily to prepare his meals
3. She has old back injury which bothers her at night if she lies on the back.	3. Turn from one side to the other during the night. Keep off her back. Watch for pressure areas on hips	3. Every hour during the night, Mrs. Johnson will be turned from side to side, keeping her off her back. No reddened areas on hips noted.
4. Poor circulation to feet	4. Have Mrs. Johnson exercise her legs at least once each shift. Keep socks on her feet at all times.	4. During the day, Mrs. Johnson's feet are warm to touch and have a pink color

Fig. 11. Problem-approach card.

"clumping," that is, of many activities being relegated to one time. By stating time and frequency in the nursing action statement the nursing care can be spaced evenly throughout the day. And, of course, there is a record of what, when, and how the care was delivered. A major benefit to writing descriptive and clear statements of the nursing actions is that it helps organize the client's treatment program and the work schedule of the staff, therefore providing for coordination and comprehensive care.

An example of the part of the nursing care plan where needs/problems and nursing approaches are stated is illustrated in Fig. 11. The nursing care plan as presented in the "scheduled-event" card (Fig. 10) and the "problem-approach" card (Fig. 11) is so designed that it could fit into the familiar hospital Kardex. One look at the schedule of daily care and the second card with the individual's problems and the nursing approaches gives the health worker a clear picture of the client's plan of care. Any item that is on the scheduled-event care card does not need to reappear on the problem-approach care card. To keep both cards functional and yet not create added busy work, the nurse will separate daily care from problem areas and periodically update both.

Evaluative criteria

The last column on the problem-approach care card (Fig. 11) is provided for an evaluative statement. Even though the nursing action statement is clearly stated, it is necessary to include a definitive evaluative statement. For to state "give pain medication by hypodermic injection 3 hours from the last injection" does not tell the nurse if the action accomplished pain relief. An evaluative statement that describes the expected outcome of the action enables the nurse to determine how the action will be evaluated.[11] For example:

> **Action:** Give pain medication by hypodermic injection every 3 hours from the last injection. Do not wait for the client to ask.
>
> **Evaluative criteria:** One-half hour after administering the pain medication by hypodermic injection the client will appear more comfortable and will state pain relief. This stage of pain relief will last at least 2 hours.

When the evaluative statement sets the limitations of expectations, the nurse is able to determine the action's effectiveness. In the above statement the nurse is attempting to evaluate the effectiveness of the pain medication and unless the expectations of the medication's action are definitively stated no documented evidence is available to justify any further action.

After a nursing action is evaluated, the nurse then decides what to do with the findings. If the action achieved the goal, it is maintained and becomes part of the permanent care plan. If the action did not achieve the desired effect, it is removed from the care plan, the situation is reassessed, and another cycle of the nursing process is begun. For instance, if in the above example the nurse discovers the pain medication is not relieving the client's pain, a whole new problem exists and a decision is warranted as to what action to take next. At the same time the nurse may have discovered new problems or needs that in turn also generate a need to consider new alternative actions. It is this recycling and reidentification of problems that makes the dynamic and ever-changing nature of the process of nursing such a challenge.

Care plans for extended care

The nursing care plans presented in Figs. 10 and 11 are designed for hospital care. The same concepts and content areas are applicable to care plans in other settings, but because the care is not on a 24-hour basis the care plans are considerably more simple. Fig. 12 is an example of a care plan that might be used by nurses in industrial settings, clinics, or for nurses who

---

[11]See Chapter Four for a detailed discussion on how to write an evaluative statement that clearly indicates an expected outcome.

provide care in the home. The nursing history card is an account of the first visit where the assessment is made. It could include many other areas of personal history depending on the agency policy and the type of care offered. The ongoing plan is recorded, evaluated, and revised on the problem-approach plan card. Each visit begins with an evaluation of the client's progress since

NURSING HISTORY

Date: Name: _____ Age: _____ Sex: _____ Single__ Married__ Divorced __ Source of Referral: _____ Occupation: _____ Allergies: _____ Medications: _____ _____ _____ **Expectations for care**	Health history Presenting health problem	Observations and comments

PROBLEM APPROACH PLAN

Date:	Observations and areas discussed	(Objectives for care) Problems or needs	Nursing approach	Evaluative criterion
Visit 2				
Visit 3				
Visit 4				

Fig. 12. Care plan for extended-care facility.

his last visit, as determined by the evaluative criteria. Again the process of identifying problems utilizing the stress-response model (Chapter Three) provides the nurse with the data necessary for planning care. Periodic summary of the problem-approach plan provides data that are then entered into the client's permanent chart as a record of his progress.

INITIATING AND REVISING THE HOSPITAL NURSING CARE PLAN

The process of preparing, implementing, and evaluating nursing care is a time-consuming activity. With an increasing number of persons seeking care and the overwhelming demands being placed on nursing staffs, it seems impossible that nurses have time to plan care. But the dynamic nature of nursing necessitates a planning process. There are several ways in which nursing personnel can plan and evaluate care even within the constraints of a busy hospital. Whether the nursing plan is designed for a hospitalized client, a person in a clinic, or for one in the home, the same planning, evaluating, and revising are necessary.

There are several times during each shift of personnel in a hospital that nurses can prepare and update the nursing care plan. Nurses can initiate and revise care plans during (1) the client admission conference, (2) the report conference, (3) the assignment conference, and (4) the client-centered case study conferences.

Initiating the hospital care plan

The nursing care plan begins when the client enters the hospital. The registered nurse admits the client and takes the nursing history. In some instances nurse's aides have been taught to conduct an admission conference. Nursing history forms that elicit pertinent data have been developed with some success. But sometime during this early phase of hospitalization the nurse will visit and welcome the client, for it is during this first encounter that the nurse-client relationship begins. During this early dialogue the nurse begins the initial assessment. How and what transpires during this conference has much to do with how the client views his illness and what he expects of his hospitalization. A major element to remember as part of the admission conference is to provide privacy. Some of the things the nurse wants to know or that the client wishes to discuss are privileged information. In some hospitals an admission nurse, whose office is in the lobby, admits the client in the quiet and secluded comfort of a friendly and cozy room. The client is then sent to the laboratory and the x-ray department for an admission work-up before he is assigned to his room. The advantage of this procedure is that the client is provided with an atmosphere of privacy and comfort while the nursing history is taken. The disadvantage is that he does not meet the nurse who will care for him until after the interview is completed. The success of this kind of procedure depends on the comprehensiveness of the history form. The nurse responsible for the client's care transcribes the pertinent data from the nursing history to the nursing care plan. After doing so, the nurse is free to visit the client to validate the admission nurse's observations and interpretations and to focus on getting to know the client. Nursing care plans that are initiated early in the nurse's contact with the client are often based on inadequate data. As the nurse and the other team members spend more time with the client, they are able to collect more information. This additional information validates and supplements the original plan and influences decisions that the nurse makes about problems and approaches. Every contact with the client results in more new data. In order that the care plan keeps abreast of the changing needs of the client, periodic conferences are needed. It is at these conferences that the staff can share their observations and new data.

Revising the care plan during the change-of-shift conference

The "report conference," or "change-of-shift conference," is an excellent time for revising or updating the care plan. It is at this time that one team reports off duty and communicates the events of their time on duty to the team coming on duty. It is an excellent time for the two groups of nursing staff to share ideas, expectations, and concern about the client they care for. The nurse reporting off gives an account of: (1) any changes in the client's condition—the current status of each client, (2) the priority problems or needs of the client, (3) the client's ability to cope with his problems, (4) the nursing goals that were met, and (5) the nursing care that was not completed.

Changes in the client's condition, his ability to cope, and his response to therapy create or alleviate nursing problems. During the change-of-shift conference the nurse reporting off duty describes any changes that have occurred and how the client is coping with these changes. Some problems that were significant and of top priority have been resolved, whereas new ones have taken their place. For example, one of the clients returning from surgery had problems stabilizing his vital signs. At the change-of-shift conference it is reported that he is maintaining stable vital signs but that he has not voided since surgery. These changing problems are reflected in the plan of care as the nurse coming on duty makes note of the new problem in the care plan. Priorities will be established and the nursing approaches modified to meet the new nursing goal.

Some of the early identified problems or needs gain clarity as more data are accrued and thus necessitate modification in the problem statement. For instance, the first contact with the client who has just been told that he has a malignant disease indicates he is frightened. However, as the nurse and the client get to know each other the nurse discovers he believes he is dying. The problem can now be stated more definitively. This in turn leads the staff to consider new alternative approaches and their consequences, value, and risk for meeting the modified problem.

The nursing care plan also changes as a result of the client's ability to cope. Consider the person with a myocardial infarction who is having difficulty accepting the restrictions on his activity. In the acute stage of his condition he is fed and bathed to conserve his energy, thus decreasing the work load on his heart. Some persons have difficulty coping with this dependent role. But as they have a chance to verbalize their feelings and to adapt to the situation, most accept assistance without resentment. Information of this nature is an important part of the nurse's report, for the goals for care will need to be revised to meet the changing needs of the client.

The statement of the client's problem is crucial to the development of effective nursing actions. It is well worth the investment of time and effort to change and update the problem statement in the care plan, if the care is to remain individualized and current.

The part of the care plan that is subject to the greatest degree of refinement is the nursing approaches. As the nurse describes the nursing actions that were tried, those that were successful, and those that did not accomplish the desired effect, it becomes evident that changes are necessary. Even the successful actions create change as the focus is shifted to other problems. For instance, the new mother who is learning to feed her baby may need repeated demonstrations and encouragement before she is able to move on to learn how to diaper, bathe, and dress the infant. If at any point along the way the mother is having difficulty, the nurse reexamines the goals for teaching, the strategies used, and revises the approach as necessary. The nursing approaches in either case are changing constantly because the nurse is either revising the present approaches to accomplish the present goal or devising new approaches to meet the new goal. Updating the care plan to include new or modified approaches is the responsibility of both the nurse reporting off duty and the nurse coming on duty. If each alters the plan as necessary and when appropriate, the plan remains a viable and functional guide for nursing action. The nurse reporting can alter the care plan during her tour of duty as changes occur. The nurse receiving the report can refine the care plan as she listens to the account of the many changes in the client's condition. Working together these nurses, as well as all those who have had contact with the client, can keep the nursing care plan current and usable.

Revising the care plan during the assignment conference

Sometime after the change of shift, the registered nurse sits down with the team and makes assignments. There are many variations of this procedure. In some agencies the assignments are posted before the conference begins. In others the nurses prefer to make nursing rounds with the team and to discuss the plan of care at the bedside with the client before making assignments. In any event at some time the team meets to discuss the plan of action for their tour of duty. It is during the assignment conference that (1) work assignments are delegated; (2) the nursing care plan is further refined; (3) the team members have a chance to increase their understanding of the client's needs, problems, and care; (4) new or "float" staff nurses are oriented to each client's plan of care. Responsibility for particular tasks is set as each client's care is delegated to specific members of the team. Before the team proceeds with their work assignment, each client's care plan is reviewed. The team scans the care plans for a review of the changes in nursing problems and any alterations in nursing actions. The team determines what the client's needs are, how each one is coping, and what actions might help them cope more efficiently. A major value of utilizing the assignment conference for reviewing the care plan for possible revision is that it provides a way of orienting new staff members or "float" personnel to the individualized needs and care of each client. It also reorients nursing staff who have been ill, on a day off, or are returning from vacation to the care of each client.

Revising the care plan during the client-centered conference

It has been said that the client-centered conference is the center of team nursing and that from this conference all team activities stem.[12] The client-centered conference, usually held sometime during the shift when most of the nursing activities have been completed, is the conference at which the team discusses its goals and evaluates the delivery of care. The client-centered conference (1) creates a team approach to decision making because it involves each member of the team in each client's plan of care; (2) encourages the pooling of resources, since every team member has a share in the decisions made about each client's care; and (3) promotes staff development. The emphasis of the client-centered conference is on evaluation; the client's needs and the nursing approaches are discussed in light of any needed changes. The conference is more than a report of what was done; it is during this conference that the nursing team presents and studies each client's problems to determine whether his needs are being met. By pooling ideas and sharing knowledge, the team members assure the client of all the benefits to be derived from the consideration given him by all members of the team. Collectively, the team members reassess each client's problems, making changes in the priority order as needed. The long-term and short-term nursing goals are reviewed and modified whenever needed. Alternative nursing actions are proposed and evaluated, with consideration given to the probability, value, and risk of their consequences. Finally, decisions are made and nursing actions are selected. All these changes are entered on the care plan.

---

[12]Kron: Nursing team leadership, p. 117.

CARE PLANS IN EXTENDED-CARE FACILITIES

The process of initiating and revising a care plan for the client in a clinic, a physician's office, in a public health agency, or in the home is much like the one utilized in the hospital. But the content of these care plans differ. Care plans in extended-care facilities (1) generally cover a longer period of time (although each separate visit does not usually last over an hour, the total time the client receives health supervision is usually longer than the time a person spends in a hospital); (2) are designed to resolve nonacute health problems; and (3) are used again and again as a resource, since the client returns to the same clinic, physician, or agency with another health problem at a later date. These differences influence the type of care plan developed. For instance, unlike persons hospitalized in an acute stage of illness, individuals seen in the home, the clinic, or the physician's office are seeking help to prevent an illness or are in a recuperative stage from an illness. Their health problems are of a rehabilitative, preventative, or minor nature.

Initiating the care plan

During the first encounter with the client, the nurse gathers data by taking a nursing history as the first step in making an assessment. Throughout the interview the nurse observes and records data about the client's attitudes concerning health, his perceptions of his health needs, and his expectations for care. The nurse encourages the client to become involved in talking out his problems, desires, and needs. The end result is the identification of his health needs. Before leaving the interview, the client and the nurse set goals and establish some means of reaching these goals. Unlike the hospital setting in which the client is often dependent on the nurse for care, the client receiving help in the extended-care facility is expected to assume major responsibility for carrying out the health plan. No nurse will be around to remind him to do his exercises, eat the correct food, or to take his medication. These activities are the responsibility of the client. So, as the care plan evolves, the client is initiated into the habit of evaluating his own needs, establishing his own goals, and activating the care plan.

Revising the care plan

At the beginning of each visit the care plan is reviewed by the nurse and the client. The nursing goals are evaluated. The client's ability to follow through on decisions, to seek help from other resources in the community, and his degree of independence are appraised. His attainment of the identified nursing goals largely depends on his ability to carry out the plan of care independently. If the evaluation reveals little or no progress, the situation is reassessed and revisions are made as needed.

Successive contacts over a period of time produce a longitudinal record of the client's progress and of the nursing actions that helped the client. Periodic analysis of these records gives the nurse and the client data for possible revision. Conferences with multidisciplinary professionals are also an excellent means of helping the nurse gain new insight into the client's problems. These conferences also contribute to the development of new approaches for care.

SUMMARY

The nursing care plan is a means of implementing the planned care. Since the care plan gives information about what nursing care is needed and how it is to be given, it is a guide for action. A nursing care plan defines the care for the individual client. It provides for continuity of care by providing information to all personnel involved in the delivery of care; everyone caring for the client has access to the care plan and is therefore able to carry out the program of individualized care. Notations of the client's needs, problems, preferences, and scheduled daily care are included to provide the client with comprehensive care.

Nursing care plans also contribute to the coordination of care. Diagnostic tests, treatments, consultations, and other activities performed by nonnursing personnel appear on the plan of care. A view of the care plan tells the nurse what will happen, when it will happen, and where it will occur.

Care plans that do not change are not useful. Revision is necessary if the care plan is to remain functional. The nursing care plan can be revised during the report conference, the assignment conference, and the client-centered conference. Since care plans make possible a more accurate assessment of the nursing care, they contribute to the development of the staff's knowledge and skill.

Planning and implementing nursing care without a care plan is like exploring a strange land without a map; without something to provide direction the venture is aimless.

Suggested readings

Contra Costa County Staff Public Health Nurses: Recording the home visit, Nurs. Outlook, February 1967, pp. 38-40.

Cornell, Sadie H., and Brush, Francis: Systems approach to nursing care plans, Amer. J. Nurs. **71**(7):1376-1378, 1971.

Hull, Edith Hollander: Nursing records of patient's operations, Amer. J. Nurs. **71**(6):1156-1157, 1971.

Lambertsen, Eleanor: Nursing care plans should reflect present and future patient needs, Mod. Hosp. **103**(4), October, 1964.

Leimo, Amelia: Planning patient centered care, Amer. J. Nurs. **52**(3), March, 1952.

Little, Dolores, and Carnevali, Doris: The nursing care planning system, Nurs. Outlook **19**(3), March, 1971.

Palisin, Helen E.: Nursing care plans are a snare and a delusion, Amer. J. Nurs. 71(1):63-66, 1971.

Perry, Jeanne H.: Written nursing care plan, Hosp. Progr. July, 1963.

Rhinehart, Elma Mae: Management of nursing care, New York, 1969, The Macmillan Company.

Toffler, Alvin: Future shock, New York, 1970, Bantam Books, Inc.

Wagner, Bernice: The nursing care plan, Nurs. Outlook 9(3), 1961.

Wood, Marion: A guide to better care—a nursing plan, Amer. J. Nurs. 61(12), 1961.

BIBLIOGRAPHY

Andrews, Priscilla, and Yankauer, Alfred: The pediatric nurse practitioner, Amer. J. Nurs. **71**(3):504-509, 1971.

Angrist, Shirley: Nursing care: the dream and the reality, Amer. J. Nurs. **65**(4):66-68, 1965.

Aquilera, Donna, Messick, Janice M., and Farrell, Marlene S.: Crisis intervention: theory and methodology, St. Louis, 1970, The C. V. Mosby Co.

Banathy, Bela H.: Instructional systems, Belmont, 1968, Fearon Publishers.

Bennis, Warren G., Beene, Kenneth D., and Chin, Robert: The planning of change: readings in the applied behavioral sciences, New York, 1962, Holt, Rinehart & Winston, Inc.

Berggken, Helen J., and Zagornik, A. Dawn: Teaching nursing process to beginning students, Nurs. Outlook **16**(7):32-35, 1968.

Besson, Gerald: The health-illness spectrum, Amer. J. Public Health **57**:1904, 1967.

Bevis, Em Olivia: Curriculum building in nursing: a process, St. Louis, The C. V. Mosby Co. (To be published in 1973.)

Bloom, B. S., and Krathwohl, P. R.: Taxonomy of educational objectives. Handbook I, Cognitive domain, New York, 1956, David McKay Co., Inc.

Brinling, Trudy: Tearing down a wall, Amer. J. Nurs. **71**(7):1406-1409, 1971.

Bross, L. D. J.: Design for decision, New York, 1953, The Macmillan Company.

Brown, Esther Lucile: Newer dimensions of patient care, part I, New York, 1961, Russell Sage Foundation.

Brown, Martha, and Fowler, Grace: Psychodynamic nursing: a biosocial orientation, ed. 4, Philadelphia, 1971, W. B. Saunders Company.

Burrill, Marjorie: Helping students identify and solve problems, Nurs. Outlook February, 1966, pp. 46-48.

Campbell, Margaret: Identifying nursing problems, Canad. Nurse, February, 1965.

Cannon, Walter B.: The wisdom of the body, New York, 1939, W. W. Norton & Co., Inc.

Caplan, Gerald: An approach to community mental health, New York, 1961, Grune & Stratton, Inc.

Cipolla, Josephine, and Collings, Gilbeart H., Jr.: Nurse clinicians in industry, Amer. J. Nurs. **71**(8):1530-1534, 1971.

Clissold, Grace K., and Metz, Edith A.: Evaluation—a tangible process, Nurs. Outlook **14**(3):41-45, 1966.

Collins, Rosella D.: Problem solving, a tool for patients, too, Amer. J. Nurs. **68**(7):1483-1485, 1968.

Defining Clinical Content, Community Health Nursing, Western Interstate Commission for Higher Education, Boulder, February 1967.

DeTornyay, Rheba, and Bergman, Abraham B.: Two views on the latest health manpower issue, Amer. J. Nurs. **71**(5):974-977, 1971.

Douglas, Laura Mae, and Bevis, Em Olivia: Team leadership in action, St. Louis, 1970, The C. V. Mosby Co.

Dunn, Halbert L.: High-level wellness, Virginia, 1961, R. W. Beatty, Ltd.

Durr, Eleanor, and Ferro, Louis E.: I.V. therapy as a nursing responsibility, RN, September, 1970, pp. 38-44.

Engle, George: Homeostasis, behavioral adjustment and the concept of health and disease. In Grinker, Roy R., editor: Mid-century psychiatry, Springfield, Ill., Charles C Thomas, Publisher, 1953.

Fact sheet, American Humanist Association, San Francisco, 1970, Humanist House.

Fast, Julius: Body language, New York, 1970, J. B. Lippincott Co.

Folta, Jeannette, and Deck, Edith S., editors: A sociological framework for patient care, New York, 1966, John Wiley & Sons, Inc.

Forum, Fall-Winter ed., 1971, J. C. Penney Co.

Fox, Madeline, J.: Talking with patients who can't answer, Amer. J. Nurs. **71**(6):1146-1149, 1971.

Francis, Gloria M.: This thing called problem solving, J. Nurs. Educ. **6**:27-30, 1967.

Freeman, Ruth B.: Community health nursing practice, Philadelphia, 1970, W. B. Saunders Company.

Gagne, Robert M.: The conditions of learning, New York, 1965, Holt, Rinehart & Winston, Inc.

Gagne, Robert M.: Educational objectives and human performance. In Learning and the educational process, Krumboltz, J. S., editor: 1965, Rand McNally & Co.

Gardner, John W.: Self-renewal, New York, 1964, Harper & Row, Publishers.

Geitgey, Doris A., and Crowley, Dorothy: Preparing objectives, Amer. J. Nurs. **65**(1):95-97, 1965.

Geitgey, Doris A.: Self-pacing: a guide to nursing care, Nurs. Outlook **17**(8):48-49, 1969.

Goerke, Lenor, and Stebbins, Ernest L.: Mustard's introduction to public health, New York, 1968, The Macmillan Company.

Hall, Jay, O'Leary, Vincent, and Williams, Martha: The decision-making grid: a model of decision-making styles, California Management Review **7**(2):43-54, 1964.

Hardiman, Margaret A.: Interviewing or social chit-chat, Amer. J. Nurs. **71**(7):1379-1381, 1971.

Hazzard, Mary Elizabeth: An overview of systems theory, Nurs. Clin. N. Amer. **6**(3):385-393, 1971.

Henderson, Virginia: The nature of nursing, New York, 1966, The Macmillan Company.

Hershey, Nathan: Profession of unlimited potential, Amer. J. Nurs. **71**(7): 1410-1412, 1971.

Hewitt, Helen E., and Pesznecker, Betty L.: Blocks to communicating with patients, Amer. J. Nurs. **64**(7):101-103, 1964.

Hofling, Charles, and Leininger, Madeleine: Basic psychiatric concepts in nursing, Philadelphia, 1967, J. B. Lippincott Co.

Isler, Charlotte: Radiation therapy—the nurse and the patient, RN, March, 1971, pp. 48-51.

Jahoda, Marie: Current concepts of positive mental health, New York, 1958, Basic Books, Inc., Publishers.

Jamann, Joann: Health is a function of ecology, Amer. J. Nurs. **71**(5):970-973, 1971.

Johnson, Miriam M.: A sociological analysis of the nurse role, Social interaction and patient care, Philadelphia, 1965, J. B. Lippincott Co., pp. 29-39.

Jordan, Judith D., and Shipp, Joseph: The primary health care professional was a nurse, Amer. J. Nurs. **71**(5):922-925, 1971.

Jourard, Sidney M.: Disclosing man to himself, Princeton, 1968, D. Van Nostrand Co.

Jourard, Sidney M.: The transparent self, Princeton, 1964, D. Van Nostrand Co.

Jude, James R., and Blam, James O.: Fundamentals of cardiopulmonary resuscitation, Phildelphia, 1965, F. A. Davis Co.

Kemp, Jerrold E.: Instructional design, Belmont, 1971, Fearon Publishers.

Kerlinger, Fred N.: Foundations of behavioral research, New York, 1965, Holt, Rinehart & Winston, Inc.

Klagsbreen, Samuel C.: Communications in the treatment of cancer, Amer. J. Nurs. **71**(5):944-948, 1971.

Komorita, Nori I.: Nursing diagnosis, Amer. J. Nurs. **63**(12):83-86, 1963.

Krathwohl, David R., Bloom, Benjamin S., and Masia, Bertram B.: Taxonomy of educational objectives: affective domain, New York, 1956, David McKay Co., Inc.

Lambertsen, Eleanor: Nursing care plan should reflect present and future patient needs, Mod. Hosp. **103**(4):128, 1964.

Langner, Thomas S., and Michael, Stanley T.: Life, stress and mental health, Vol. II, London, 1963, The Free Press of Glencoe.

Lewis, Garland K.: Communication, a factor in meeting emotional crisis, Nurs. Outlook **13**:36-39, 1965.

Lunberg, George, Schog, Clarence, and Larsen, Otto: Sociology, New York, 1963, Harper & Row, Publishers.

MacDonald, Frederick: Educational psychology, ed. 2, Belmont, 1969, Wadsworth Publishing Co., Inc.

MacDonald, Frederick J., and Harms, Mary T.: Theoretical model for an experimental curriculum, Nurs. Outlook, **14**(8):48-51, 1966.

Mager, Robert F.: Developing attitude toward learning, Belmont, 1968, Fearon Publishers.

Mager, Robert F.: Preparing instructional objectives, Palo Alto, 1962, Fearon Publishers.

Mann, J. George: Future hospitals will go where the people are, Mod. Hosp. **110**(6):84-89, 1968.

Mansfield, Elaine: Care plans to stimulate learning, Amer. J. Nurs. **68**(12):2592-2593, 1968.

Maslow, Abraham H.: Toward a psychology of being, ed. 2, Princeton, 1962, D. Van Nostrand Co.

Mathwig, Gean: Nursing science, the theoretical core of nursing knowledge, Image **4**(1):20-23, 1970.

May, Rollo, editor: Existential psychology, New York, 1960, Random House, Inc.

May, Rollo: Love and will, New York, 1969, W. W. Norton & Company, Inc.

McCabe, Grace: Cultural influences on patient behavior, Amer. J. Nurs. **60**(8):1101-1104, 1960.

Meldman, Monte, Newman, Cernard, Scholler, Donna, and Peterson, Paul: Patients' responses to nurse-psychotherapists, Amer. J. Nurs. **71**(6):1150-1151, 1971.

Mereness, Dorothy: Essentials of psychiatric nursing, ed. 8, St. Louis, 1970, The C. V. Mosby Co.

Nightingale, Florence: Notes on nursing, London, 1859, Harris & Sons.

Parsons, Talcott: On becoming a person, the social system, New York, 1964, The Free Press of Glencoe.

Peplau, Hildegard E.: Talking with patients, Amer. J. Nurs. **60**(7):964-966, 1960.

Perry, Jeanne H.: Written nursing care plan, Hosp. Progr. **63**:71-73, 80, 1963.

P.N.A.–threat or boon to pediatricians? RN **34**(6):70-71, 1971.

Rae, Nancy Mara: Caring for patients following open heart surgery, Amer. J. Nurs. **63**(11):77-82, 1963.

Reves, Ruth E.: Priorities according to needs, In Stewart, D. M., and Vincent, P. A., editors: Public Health Nursing, Iowa, 1968, William C. Brown Company, Publishers.

Robischon, Paulette: Community nursing in a changing climate, Nurs. Outlook **19**(6):410-413, 1971.

Robischon, Paulette, and Scott, Diane: Role theory and its application in family nursing, Nurs. Outlook **17**(7):52-53, 1969.

Rodgers, Carl: On becoming a person, Boston, 1961, Houghton Mifflin Company.

Rogers, Martha E.: Educational revolution in nursing, New York, 1961, The Macmillan Company.

Ruesch, Jurgen: Disturbed communication, New York, 1957, W. W. Norton & Company, Inc.

Ruesch, Jurgen: Therapeutic communication, New York, 1961, W. W. Norton & Company, Inc.

Ruesch, Jurgen: The observer & the observed: human communication theory, Toward a Unified Theory of Human Behavior, New York, 1956, Basic Books, Inc., Publishers, pp. 36-54.

Schachter, S.: Deviation, rejection and communication, J. Abnorm. Psychol. **46**:190-207, 1951.

Schweer, Mildred E., and Gardella, Frances A.: Planning, orienting and preparing for a new kind of nurse leadership, Nurs. Outlook **18**(5):42-16, 1970.

Selye, Hans: The stress syndrome, Amer. J. Nurs. **65**:97-99, 1965.

Selye, Hans: The stress of life, New York, 1956, McGraw-Hill Book Co.

Shetland, Margaret: Teaching and learning, Amer. J. Nurs. **65**(9):112-116, 1965.

Shostrom, Everett L.: Man, the manipulator, New York, 1967, Bantam Books, Inc.

Simmons, Janet A.: The nurse-patient relationship in psychiatric nursing, Philadelphia, 1969, W. B. Saunders & Company.

Smith, Dorothy: Writing objectives as a nursing practice skill, Amer. J. Nurs. **71**(2):319-320, 1971.

Smuts, J. C.: Holism and evolution, New York, 1926, The Macmillan Company.

Stevens, Leonard F.: Nurse-patient discussion groups, Amer. J. Nurs. **63**(12):67-69, 1963.

Stewart, I. M.: Possibilities of standardization in nursing techniques, Mod. Hosp., June 1919.

Straus, David, and others: Tools for change, ed. 2, San Francisco, 1971, Interaction Associates, Inc.

Tyler, Ralph W.: Some persistent questions on the defining of objectives, In Lindvall, C. M., editor: Defining Educational Objectives, Pittsburgh, 1964, University of Pittsburgh Press.

Ungvarski, Peter: Mechanical stimulation of coughing, Amer. J. Nurs. **71**(12):2358-2361, 1971.

Wagner, Berniece M.: Care plans right, reasonable and reachable, Amer. J. Nurs. **69**(5):986-990, 1969.

Walker, Elizabeth: Primex—the family nurse practitioner program, Nurs. Outlook **20**(1):28-31, 1972.

Wandelt, Mabel: Guide for the beginning researcher, New York, 1970, Appleton-Century-Crofts.

Wason, Edna: A team leader's day, Amer. J. Nurs. **55**(4):1470-1471, 1955.

Wesseling, Elizabeth: The adolescent facing amputation, Amer. J. Nurs. **65**(1):91-94, 1965.

Wiedenbach, Ernestine: The helping art of nursing, Amer. J. Nurs. **63**(11):54-57, 1963.

Wolff, Harold G.: Stress and disease, Springfield, Ill., 1952, Charles C Thomas, Publisher.

Wood, Marion: A guide to better care—a nursing plan, Amer. J. Nurs. **61**(12):61, 1961.

Index